PACK OF THIEVES?

52 FEMALE FACTORY LIVES

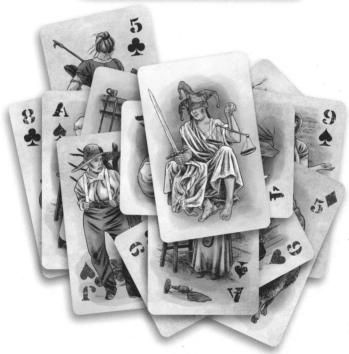

PORT
ARTHUR
HISTORIC
SITES

© Port Arthur Historic Site Management Authority, 2014.
This work is copyright. Apart from any use as permitted
under the Copyright Act of 1968 and its amendments, no
part of this book may be reproduced, stored in a retrieval
system or transmitted by any means or process whatsoever
without prior permission of the publisher. Published by:
Port Arthur Historic Site Management Authority, Arthur
Highway, Port Arthur, Tasmania, 7182, Australia.

Websites: http://www.portarthur.org.au,
and http://www.femalefactory.org.au

Design: Poco People.

Printed in Australia by Monotone
Art Printers Pty Ltd, Hobart.

National Library of Australia
Cataloguing-in-Publication entry:

Title: Pack of thieves?:52 female factory lives.
ISBN: 9780957939462 (paperback)
Notes: Includes bibliographical references.

Subjects: Cascades Female Factory (Tas.)—History.
Women convicts—Tasmania—History—19th century.
Women prisoners—Tasmania—History—19th century.
Convict labor—Tasmania—History—19th century.
Port Arthur (Tas.)—History—19th century.

Other Authors/Contributors: Port Arthur Historic Site
Management Authority (Tas.), issuing body.
Dewey Number:365.4309946

The *Cascades Female Factory women — through image and
stories* project is supported through funding from the
Australian Government's *Your Community Heritage Grants
Programme, 2012-2013.*

Reprinted 2014

CONTENTS

ACKNOWLEDGEMENTS

This has been an exciting project involving a number of people, first and foremost the steering committee including Port Arthur Historic Site Management Authority staff: Robyn Bradshaw, Dr Jane Harrington, Susan Hood, Greta McDonald and Dr Jody Steele, and members of the Female Convicts Research Centre: Dr Lucy Frost, Colette McAlpine and Dr Dianne Snowden, all of whom are also members of the Cascades Female Factory Community Advisory Committee. Writers include a number of the steering committee, as well as a contribution by Dr Alison Alexander—all contributions have been greatly appreciated and we have all learned a lot about the women within these pages. To Simon Barnard for his wit, professionalism and most importantly his interpretation of the women that inspired the artwork for the playing cards as well as the map in the book—the images are truly wonderful! To Dr Trudy Cowley for her initial assistance in helping us select some of the characters, and providing assistance with, and access to the Female Convicts in Van Diemen's Land database, as well as contributing text for the glossary. A big thank you to Jemma Sims, a Cascades Female Factory Historic Site volunteer who located the convict record links for us and saved us some time, and to Jane Harrington for her proof reading. To Poco People for designing the book, and Monotone Art Printers for continuing to work with us on this second version of the Pack of thieves books. And finally, our appreciation to the Australian Government and the Your Community Heritage Grants Programme for making this project possible.

All successful projects need a good leader, and in this case we acknowledge the skills and endeavours of our Project Manager, Susan Hood. She steered us on a straight path and provided the right nudges at the right time. Resistance was futile! Thank you Susan.

As with the Port Arthur version of Pack of thieves, although we have conducted a thorough research of all the records that have been immediately available to us, there are many other resources that due to the time constraints we have not been able to consult. We would welcome further information on any of the convicts and civil officers within this publication and would be delighted to hear from their descendants. The work owes much to the research of the writers, and all mistakes are of our own making.

CONTRIBUTORS' BIOGRAPHIES

ALISON ALEXANDER has written 24 books about Tasmanian history, ranging from biographies to commissioned histories of a variety of institutions and areas. She completed her PhD in 1991 on 'The public role of women in Tasmania 1803-1914' and has been employed by the University of Tasmania as tutor, casual lecturer, and editor of *The Companion to Tasmanian History*. Alison published *Governor's ladies: the wives and mistresses of Tasmania's Governors* in 1987, followed in 2010 by *Tasmania's convicts: how felons built a free society*, and more recently *The ambitions of Jane Franklin* in 2013. She has been involved with numerous historical societies as well as the Female Convicts Research Centre (FCRC) and Convict Women's Press, and she is also on the committee of the Tasmanian Historical Research Association.

SIMON BARNARD was born and grew up in Launceston. He spent a lot of time in the bush as a boy, which led to an interest in Tasmanian history. A Van Diemonian who effected a successful escape from the colony, he is an illustrator and a collector of colonial artefacts. He now lives in Melbourne with his girlfriend and a little dog 'Tuco Benedicto Pacifico Juan Maria Ramirez', also known as 'The Rat'.

LUCY FROST is Emeritus Professor of English at the University of Tasmania. Her research has focussed on the experiences of the convict women and their children transported to Van Diemen's Land during the first half of the 19th century. She is the President of the FCRC, and has been involved in the Research Centre's publications on the Launceston, Ross and Cascades Female Factories. She co-edited *Chain letters: narrating convict lives* in 2001, and her biographical study of women convicted in the courts of Scotland, *Abandoned women: exiled beyond the seas* was published in 2012.

JANE HARRINGTON has been the Director of Conservation and Infrastructure with the Port Arthur Historic Site Management Authority since 2006. She has worked in cultural heritage for more than 20 years, completing her doctoral research in 2004. She was closely involved with the contribution from the Port Arthur Historic Sites to the Australian Convict Sites World Heritage listing and subsequent management and is a member of the Australian Convict Sites Steering Committee. She now knows a lot more about female convict history than she did before this project.

SUSAN HOOD has been involved with convict records at the Port Arthur Historic Site for more years than she can recall. She manages the Resource Centre at Port Arthur and coordinates the project to identify the convicts who passed through the settlement between 1830 and 1877. She has co-authored two publications related to convicts who passed through Port Arthur: *Caught in the act: unusual offences of Port Arthur convicts* in 1999 and *Pack of thieves? 52 Port Arthur lives* in 2001. But she is pleased to have been able to assist anyone descended from a convict who seeks to interpret their ancestor's records through writing *Transcribing Tasmanian convict records* in 2003 – a 'dummy's guide' by any other name!

COLETTE MCALPINE is a database manager for the Female Convicts Research Centre. She recruits, trains and supports the FCRC volunteers, many of whom live interstate and overseas and is a passionate advocate for acknowledging the lives of the female convicts. Happy to transcribe convict records and research the lives of convict women in her spare time, including her own convict ancestors, she has contributed to a number of publications produced by Research Tasmania, and the FCRC through the Convict Women's Press.

DIANNE SNOWDEN is a professional historian and genealogist. She is founder and convenor of the Friends of the Orphan Schools, St John's Park Precinct, and as an Honorary Research Associate at the University of Tasmania is working on a longitudinal study of children admitted to the Orphan Schools, especially those who arrived free with convict parents. She completed her doctorate at the University of Tasmania in 2005 about Irish women who committed arson in order to be transported to Van Diemen's Land.

JODY STEELE - When Indiana Jones' *Raiders of the Lost Ark* was first released Jody was just four years of age, watching the film the following year along with *Star Wars – A New Hope* left her with only one choice, become a Princess of Alderaan or an archaeologist. Archaeology won and Jody received her doctorate in 2007. She then went into the world of heritage conservation and interpretation working across the state of Tasmania with the Parks and Wildlife Service and more recently having hung up her trowel, with the Port Arthur Historic Site Management Authority as Heritage Programs Manager.

PREFACE

This publication and the associated pack of playing cards has been funded by a grant under the *Sharing Community Heritage Stories* sub-programme of the *Your Community Heritage Grants Programme*, *2012-2013*, nationally funded through the (now) Commonwealth Department of the Environment. One of a number of successful projects in this category, the aim is to explore and communicate stories that connect communities with their past. The Port Arthur Historic Site Management Authority (PAHSMA) is grateful for this funding and welcomes the opportunity to provide this insight into the women historically associated with the Cascades Female Factory.

The Cascades Female Factory in Hobart is one of eleven sites in the Australian Convict Sites World Heritage listing. PAHSMA was privileged to be given management responsibility for the Cascades Female Factory Historic Site in South Hobart in 2011. The Authority also manages the Port Arthur Historic Site and the Coal Mines Historic Site on the Tasman Peninsula, both of which are also part of the Australian Convict Sites World Heritage Property. In the listing, the Female Factory is recognised as a testament to the survival and prosperity of the colonies for the benefit of Britain through the efforts of female convicts, not only through their labour, but also their post-convict success and families. Often these tales of prosperity and success go unheard. It is only through the stories of individual people that this significance can be understood today. We are proud to be able to present 52 of these stories in this volume.

PAHSMA's formal involvement with the Cascades Female Factory follows a proud legacy of management and care by the Female Factory Historic Site Ltd and the Tasmanian Parks and Wildlife Service, and the endeavours of multitudes of women and men who recognised the importance of this historic site and fought to have it protected and brought into public ownership. This more modern history of the site spans multiple decades and is yet another set of stories to be told, perhaps in a future volume. In the interim I would like to acknowledge the efforts of those who have worked so hard to protect this significant heritage place and its contribution to the history of Australia and Australians, and those who continue to labour to this end today.

I hope you find inspiration in the stories that follow.

Prof. Sharon Sullivan AO
Chair PAHSMA Board

INTRODUCTION

British transportation to Australia was the world's first conscious attempt to build a new society on the labour of convicted prisoners. Around 166,000 men, women and children were transported to Australia between 1787 and 1868, some 75,000 individuals to Van Diemen's Land. Most convicts were transported from Britain but several thousand were also shipped from Canada, America, Bermuda and other British colonies.

It is believed that some 13,000 female convicts came to Van Diemen's Land during the period 1803 to 1853 and current research suggests that over 6000 of those spent some time within the walls of the Cascades Female Factory, one of five such institutions that operated across the island. These establishments often served many purposes: as a prison, place of punishment, labour hiring depot, nursery, lying-in hospital for pregnant female convicts, workplace and temporary housing for female convicts until they were 'married' or assigned as domestic servants to free settlers or colonial officers. The Female House of Correction, colloquially known as the 'Cascades Female Factory' or just 'the Female Factory' operated between 1828 and 1856.

Following their arrival in the colony, women sent to the Female Factory were bound by the strict regulations of the institution. When the gates closed behind them, the women were cut off from the outside world. Not only had they lost family and friends, but were about to lose all of their worldly possessions, and possibly even their hair.

The women could be placed in one of three distinct classes: those assigned to hired service if well behaved, those guilty of minor offences and serving a period of punishment or whose bad conduct had improved, and those of the 'Crime Class' convicted of major offences in the colony or on board ship to the colony and suffering more extreme punishment.

Women under punishment in the Factory could be employed in a variety of tasks such as sewing, mending and laundering clothes and linen for up to ten hours a day in summer, not only a service for government establishments, but also for free settlers (providing income for the Factory). Another task was oakum picking, which involved picking the fibres of rope away from a salty tar crust so that they could be reused as caulking in ships—a task extremely harsh on the fingers of the women, especially in the cold conditions. In addition solitary confinement for days at a time on bread and water was a frequent sentence for the worst behaved convicts.

From opening its gates in late 1828, the Factory always struggled to accommodate the growing number of transportees and reoffenders and as such the site developed in a reactionary manner, responding to the many complaints of overcrowding and the subsequent conditions. Standing out the front today, the individual yards are numbered in order of construction date and not conventionally from left to right. Yard 1 (in the middle) as the name suggests was the first, originally built by Thomas Yardley Lowes in 1824 as a distillery and converted into the Factory by the end of 1828. Yard 2 (1832) was smaller than the first and took over two and a half years to construct, the northern and southern walls were lined with solitary cells, washtubs and drying lines filled the yard space and washing sheds lined the east and west walls.

Work began on the separate apartments (Yard 3) in December 1842 and one third of the new cells were occupied by mid-1844. The dimensions of this yard were similar to that of Yard 1, a number of offices were built along the southern wall and two long double-storeyed cell blocks divided the yard into three sections. Each cell block housed 28 cells on both floors making a total of 112 cells, each 4 feet six inches by 12 feet.

With Cascades being well over capacity and the conditions and infant death rates drawing much public attention in the 1840s, a number of other sites were established to take the pressure off the Factory. Women were held at a nursery site in Dynnyrne, and on board the convict hulk the *Anson*; some were moved to hiring depots and to other female factories at Ross and Launceston. Despite various locations being trialled as alternatives to Cascades the infant death rate was not improving so in an attempt to alleviate the problem and re-centralise the convict administration of females, plans were prepared in mid-1849 for a nursery—in the new Yard 4. A large nursery building ran along the western wall in this yard, with windows and a verandah facing east to capture much of the daily sun. The building was designed to house 88 women and 150 children, allowing for babies to stay with their mothers until they were weaned and placed in the care of other nursing mothers. They remained here until admitted to the Queen's Orphan School at 3 years of age. The yard also hosted a commodious cookhouse/laundry and a shelter shed was located in the centre of the large exercise yard.

The fifth or western-most yard was completed during 1852, the year before convict transportation ceased to the colony. This yard, unlike the adjacent yards, had a wall of only 5 feet surrounding it. A two-storey structure running along the eastern wall was designed to house pass-holders or probationers awaiting employment. The building was used as a dormitory and mess hall and was intended to replace the Hiring Depot at the Brickfields in New Town.

By August 1864 there were only 116 women and 29 children at the Factory—less than the first few months of its operation. The convict era was undoubtedly coming to an end and on 1 January 1865 all the Female Factory staff were transferred over to the Colonial Government. The Factory finally closed in 1877. In the years that followed the site was utilised as a male invalid depot, a female invalid depot and a boys' reformatory, and later a contagious diseases hospital, lying-in home and hospital for the insane. The complex was subdivided and in 1905 auctioned by the government to private buyers. Since then nearly all the buildings have been demolished, with a number of industrial buildings constructed across the site including a winery, marine-service boat shed, paint and fudge factory.

In the early 1970s the Women's Electoral Lobby sought out Federal government grant money for the purchase of Yard 1, handing over management to the Parks and Wild-life Service. Between 1999 and 2004 the Female Factory Historic Site Ltd acquired Yard 3 and the Matron's Quarters. And finally, in 2008, the Tasmanian State Government purchased the remaining part of Yard 4 to form the Historic Site as it is today.

Australia's convict heritage has taken on greater meaning to descendants of convicts in recent years, in particular the lives of the convict women. The passion shown by local volunteers and descendants of those with links to the Cascades Female Factory in Hobart is highly significant and growing. The modern history of the Site reflects a passionate engagement by many members of the community, both locally and more broadly. The interest has been exemplified by lobbying to obtain funds and to purchase the various yards, and the use of the Site by community groups as a forum for events and activities, as well as the long history of working with volunteers. Much of this is based on a desire to know more about the women associated with the Female Factory.

Pack of thieves? 52 Female Factory lives has taken information gathered from Tasmanian convict records and other associated sources, to recount the lives of 52 women and female staff who were incarcerated or worked at the Cascades Female Factory—the associated pack of cards provides a visual interpretation of the women based on information gleaned from their records. Composed by a number of writers, each with their own style, and in a similar vein to Port Arthur's successful *Pack of Thieves? 52 Port Arthur lives*, it aims to give a voice to 52 of the Factory's varied characters introducing the reader to the lives of those associated with this fascinating World Heritage site. Those who journeyed from faraway lands to the remote site at the base of Mt Wellington include several of the administrators who played a pivotal role in the management of the convict population. The human element of the Site's history is revealed by the individual characters in these stories, albeit a small representation of the thousands of women who served sentences within the walls of the Female Factory. Whether you are a descendant or just have an interest in the Site and the women who spent time here, you will find something of interest in the following pages.

Susan Hood and Jody Steele
Port Arthur Historic Site
Management Authority

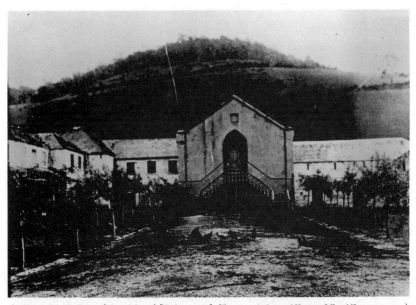

The Chapel, Cascades Factory (Women's Prison) [Yard 1, c1900]. (Tasmanian Archive and Heritage Office, NS 1013-1-1757)

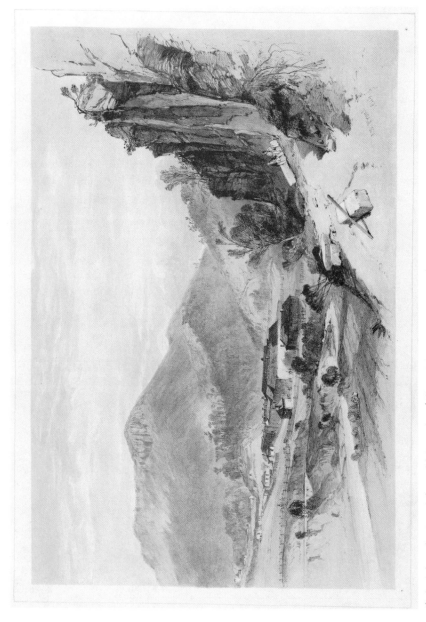

The female factory from Proctor's Quarry. J.S. Prout, 1844. (Allport Library and Museum of Fine Arts, Tasmanian Archive and Heritage Office, AUTAS001139586879)

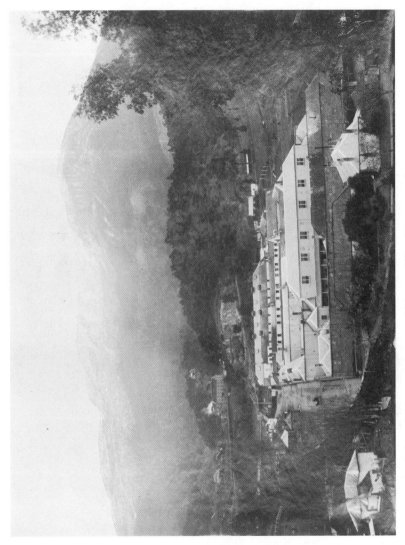

Female Factory, Cascades [c1900]. (Tasmanian Archive and Heritage Office, NS 1013-1-45)

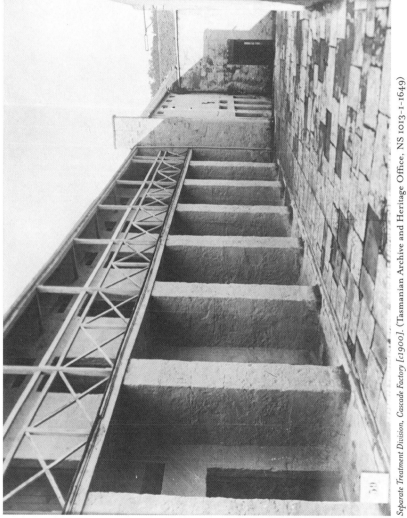

14

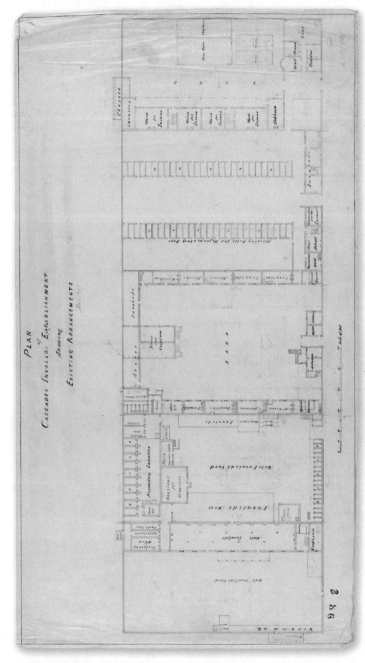

Plan of Cascades Invalid Establishment showing existing arrangements, May 1877. (Tasmanian Archive and Heritage Office, PWD 266-1-410)

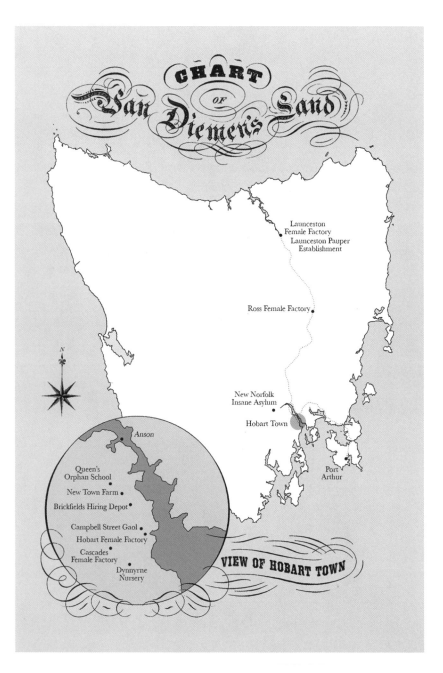

CHART *OF* Van Diemen's Land

Launceston
Female Factory
Launceston Pauper
Establishment

Ross Female Factory

New Norfolk
Insane Asylum

Hobart Town

Port
Arthur

Anson

Queen's
Orphan School
New Town Farm
Brickfields Hiring Depot
Campbell Street Gaol
Hobart Female Factory
Cascades
Female Factory
Dynnyrne
Nursery

VIEW OF HOBART TOWN

MARY
DERRICK

The young Mary Derrick had drifted from her faith, doing time for vagrancy and having very sticky fingers! On two separate occasions prior to appearing in the Lancaster Quarter Sessions in July 1848, she had managed to 'acquire' a pair of trousers and watch and as a result served five and a half months. It was in July 1848 that Mary was charged with stealing wearing apparel from Mrs Ann Williams, of Arrad Street, Liverpool, and sentenced to seven years transportation.

Arriving in Hobart on board the *Baretto Junior* on 25 July 1850 and recorded as just sixteen years of age, Mary must have been only fourteen when she was sentenced to the other side of the world. A Roman Catholic nurse maid from Belfast, she listed only her father John and sister Ann as relatives at home. Standing just 4 feet 11 inches with blue eyes and a fresh but slightly freckled complexion, it would appear that Mary was quite the mischievous teen.

Her rebellious streak presented like all good teenage rebels starting with disorderly conduct in both April and May of 1851 reported by Mr Pearce, the Overseer and Crime Class Constable. These two discretions earned her three weeks of separate treatment. Prone to a chat, Mary on five separate occasions was charged with offences related to talking or making noise. For talking in the dormitory, Mary lost the ability to be hired for a fortnight in August 1851. Now, at seventeen years of age, it seemed she could not let a month pass without breaking the rules.

Two offences in one day was Mary's personal best, her first, for 'knitting improperly' and the Night Officer, Mr Dennin, reported Mary for disorderly conduct that evening. For her efforts that day in September 1851, she was sentenced to the 'wash tub', with three days in solitary confinement and an additional seven days of separate treatment. Disorderly conduct, neglecting her work and a 'breach of regulations' reported by the Superintendent rounded out 1851 and gave Mary more time in separate treatment and two weeks of 'cleaning the yard'.

In a place where silence was so heavily valued, being a chatterbox inevitably resulted in punishment. In 1852 Mary received 48 hours on bread and water for 'loud talking at work', another three days on the lowly diet plus ten days at the washtub for making noise in the hospital yard. For talking in the separate apartments, it was seven days wearing punishment dress and not being allowed to exercise. In the same year, Mary was also found to have tobacco in her possession twice and was charged with the offence of 'having two aprons'—presumably not her own.

With a new year came new hope that Mary might enter her adult years with a Ticket of Leave, allowing her to work for whomever she chose and with a new level of freedom. Receiving her Ticket of Leave on 5 April 1853, she did not maintain her freedom of employment long, just three months later being charged with being a 'common prostitute' and sentenced to four months hard labour in July. By 25 October 1853 Mary's Ticket of Leave had been revoked and as a result of her prior indiscretions she was no longer to be allowed into service anywhere south of Oatlands.

Between receiving her Ticket and having it revoked, Mary applied to marry James Regan, also a transportee, on 22 August 1853, but there is no evidence that this union was ever approved or took place. In the August of 1853, James was in-between serving time in solitary for being drunk and absent from his abode and being drunk and assaulting a constable. Perhaps the officials thought Mary

could do better than the 28-year-old convict labourer with a penchant for liquor.

As much as being a chatterbox was more often than not a breach of regulations, so was sleeping in, which was reported as the offence of 'not out of bed at regular hours'. For this offence in August 1853 Mary was to spend 48 hours in the Female Factory punishment ward, again on bread and water. In November, for using obscene language, she received another month in hard labour.

The close of 1853 saw an end to Mary's rebellious behaviour, perhaps it was because she was growing out of her teenage years, or perhaps it was the influence of a good man? In mid-1854 she applied for permission to marry Francis Nicholas and at the same time received her Ticket of Leave again.

In August that same year Mary and Francis tied the knot in the Church of England in Perth (Tasmania). Francis was recorded as a 40-year-old bachelor, Mary a 19-year-old Ticket of Leave spinster. Within 37 weeks of marriage, Mary gave birth to their first son, Joseph Nicholas in Longford.

Francis and Mary went on to have at least five children, but little else is known about their lives other than they obviously resided around Campbell Town throughout the 1860s and early 1870s as that was where all the children's births were registered.

Mary's death was recorded just two days before Christmas in 1885.

MARY ANN
WOOD

'A reputed bad character with a violent temper' was how the surgeon on board the *Tory* described 19-year-old Mary Ann Wood upon her arrival into Hobart on 4 July 1845. The 5 feet 1 inch unmarried house maid from London, according to her conduct record, chose not to live up to her Roman Catholic values. She was transported for ten years for stealing apparel in the infamous Horsemonger Lane—home to the County of Surrey's main prison and it appears that Mary Ann was no stranger to the prison system. Not only was she caught stealing near one, prior to her transportation she had spent a total of eight months behind bars, two of those for stealing a hearth rug, the remaining six for stealing a shawl.

Leaving England, Mary Ann farewelled her mother Johannah, and siblings Charles, John, Ellen and Julia, all identified by the surname Herring. Perhaps some of her dozen tattoos were reminders of her family?

One tattoo was described as 'J.P. Head', which leads one to wonder if that was a tattoo of her defacto partner Job Pressley who Mary Ann declared she had lived with for four years prior to her arrest. Although the meaning of her tattoos and why she went by a different surname may remain a mystery, what we do know about Mary Ann is that she could read and write, she had a lisp and the 19-year-old brunette with a long nose and hazel eyes was determined to buck the system.

Van Diemen's Land was in the throes of implementing the Probation System, a system of staged reform when Mary Ann arrived. The system encouraged those within it to better themselves in order to gain privileges, a class system based on your crime and subsequent behaviour. In physical form, this system had resulted in the construction of a new yard inside the Cascades Female Factory—Yard 3—containing 112 separate apartments. These apartments were small solitary cells measuring about 3.5 metres long by 1.3 metres wide, and were large enough for a bed during the evening and to work at spinning, carding or sewing during the day. The idea was to separate the women from each other, in the hope of encouraging reflection, in addition to keeping those with a chance to reform away from the hardened reoffender.

It seems that Mary Ann got to know the separate apartments quite well. Less than twelve months into her sentence, on 1 May 1846, while being held on the *Anson* hulk, Mary Ann chose to disobey orders and was sentenced to four months hard labour in the separate apartments. Within two months of returning to the *Anson* she was disorderly in her ward and again returned to the Factory, this time for four months hard labour.

Eight months to reflect did not have the desired effect as after less than two months back on the *Anson* she was charged with misconduct using threatening language and sentenced this time to six months hard labour. The to and fro continued, as between 2 February and 22 December 1848 Mary Ann was sentenced to a total of ten months hard labour and an additional 24 days in solitary confinement. One stint in solitary was awarded for 'concealing herself to avoid going to chapel'. During this time Mary Ann was returned to the Factory from service by her master for being absent without leave. Her master was listed as Coverdale, perhaps Dr John Coverdale—a well known medical practitioner of the day who operated a private practice, was Deputy Registrar of births, deaths and marriages, coroner and magistrate.

Interestingly, in this instance, Mary Ann was only reprimanded and sent back to the Factory—not punished.

The following two years saw little change in her behaviour, being twice absent without leave resulting in another three months hard labour, and while at the Brickfields Hiring Depot in October 1849 she was charged with improperly having a shift in her possession that was the property of her mistress, receiving another nine months hard labour. Making use of indecent language and being in a ward without permission also made the offence list.

Talking in her separate apartment, insolence, being disorderly at Chapel, not performing her work, having a dirty apartment, exchanging petticoats and going to hospital under false pretences all appear as offences in Mary Ann's rap sheet for 1851 and 1852. Not proceeding to the depot and absenting herself from service only to be found in the hut drinking with the men and insolence are the final offences listed against her. Her last offence saw Mary Ann issued another month of hard labour, at the end of which she appears to have been hired from the Ross Female Factory.

Mary Ann's conduct record suggests that she made an application to marry John Pankhurst in July 1853, which was recommended on 14 September, and she was listed as married on 20 September, just six days later, however no record of the union can be found outside of that document. John too was a transportee, sentenced to Life he was 27 when he arrived in Van Diemen's Land in 1843. Despite being blind in one eye, the surgeon on board the *Gilmore* (3) described him as 'useful on deck' and with little of note on his record, it appears John received his Conditional Pardon in August 1854.

On 31 July 1854 Mary Ann was Free by Servitude and appears to have reformed, as there is no obvious record of her either in the convict system or local newspapers. Whether she and her husband moved interstate, or just chose to live the quiet life, we may never know.

BRIDGET
HEHIR

Red-haired Bridget Hehir was twenty when tried in County Clare, Ireland, on 28 October 1850 for cow stealing and sentenced to transportation for ten years. This was the second time Bridget was charged for stealing a cow. The first time she was sentenced to imprisonment for six months but was discharged.

Bridget, a country servant, sailed on the *Blackfriar*, arriving

in Hobart on 29 May 1851. During the voyage her behaviour was recorded as 'quiet'. She had also been quiet in gaol while waiting to be transported. In common with many of the Irish convict women, she was single, Roman Catholic and illiterate.

Initially placed in the House of Correction and then the Brickfields Hiring Depot waiting to be assigned, she did not get off to a good start in Van Diemen's Land. Less than three months after arriving in the colony, she absconded from her master and in December 1851 was returned to the House of Correction to serve six months hard labour. Bridget was pregnant at the time—and almost twelve months to the day from the time she arrived in Van Diemen's Land, she gave birth prematurely to a son Richard at the Female House of Correction. Richard Hehir lived only six days, dying on 25 May 1852. Bridget was later sent to the Queen's Orphan School as a nurse, which may have been very difficult after her own tragedy.

In March 1853 she was back in the House of Correction, most likely waiting assignment. Assigned to her new mistress in Macquarie Street in August, by October she was re-assigned to another employer, in Church Street, but three days later was back in the House of Correction briefly, and then assigned to an employer in Liverpool Street. In May 1854 Bridget was charged with insolence and refusing to work, and sentenced to four months hard labour. Things did not appear to be going well for her.

On St Patrick's Day 1855, she was sentenced to one month hard labour for using abusive language. Despite this offence, she was granted a Ticket of Leave later that month, and then recommended for a Conditional Pardon in December 1855, which was approved on 25 November 1856. She received her Free Certificate on 29 October 1860—on completion of her transportation sentence.

Bridget had four applications to marry, including two to John Poolman. The first, to Francis Lewis, was in February 1854 but Bridget had to remain free from offence for six months. The first application to John Poolman was in September 1855, and they were told they could apply again in October. When they reapplied in November 1855, the marriage was approved and gazetted but no marriage took place. Perhaps Bridget decided that fellow-convict John Appleby, a house painter, was a better option. Their marriage was approved in February 1856 and the ceremony took place on 10 March 1856 in St George's Church of England at Battery Point.

Bridget and John had at least six children, all born in Hobart between 1856 and 1866. The first, John Anthony Appleby, born in November 1856, was just over eighteen months old when he died of croup. Another son, Frederick, died at nineteen months in April 1866 from 'diarrhoea and effusion into the head'. For the birth registrations of her children, Bridget's name varied and she seems to have adopted Elizabeth as her given name about this time. Her variously adopted names saw her known as Elizabeth Eyre (1856), Elizabeth Hare (1858, 1862), Elizabeth Heir (1861) and Eliza Heir (1866).

In May 1867 Bridget was bitten by a large black snake in St David's Cemetery when she went there to visit the grave of her child. Plied with brandy, champagne, ammonia and other stimulants she eventually recovered!

Despite her marriage, she continued to display unsettled behaviour, with periodic appearances in the Police Court for minor offences. In October 1868 she was fined 5 shillings for disturbing the peace. However the tipping point for Bridget came in July 1871 when her husband, John Appleby, was sentenced to six years hard labour for felony (burglary), leaving her to care for her young children.

With John sent to Port Arthur, Bridget struggled to keep her family together. In August 1871 she applied to have her ten-year-old son, John, admitted to the Industrial School in Lansdowne Crescent because she was not able to maintain him. He was sent to the Boys' Home for four years. Later that month, Bridget applied to have her daughter Ann, aged 11, admitted to the Industrial School for Girls in Murray Street. She was admitted for three years. Three other children were admitted to the Queen's Asylum for Destitute Children as the Orphan School was then known. Henry aged three and Sarah aged five, were admitted in November 1871. Mary Ann aged three was admitted in August the following year. The girls remained there until May 1879 when the institution closed, at which time they were then sent to the Girls' Industrial School. Henry, who was flogged in the institution, was apprenticed out in July 1876.

In October 1871 Bridget was charged with begging alms in Battery Point. In the Hobart Police Court she stated that she had no government assistance since her husband was sent to Port Arthur and that 'the only boots she had were an old worn out pair'. She said that she had gone to the Battery Point houses simply to ask for a pair of boots. Rejecting claims that she received full rations from the Benevolent Society, 'I only get a bit of dry bread for the children', she was accused of being a drunkard and sent to gaol for one month.

In November 1871, with another woman, Catherine Sheridan, she was fined 40 shillings or two months imprisonment, for using obscene language in a public street on a Saturday night. Both women were described as 'notorious offenders'.

Having served just over two years of a six year sentence at Port Arthur, by September 1873 John was transferred to the House of Correction in Hobart, and eighteen months later the Governor remitted the residue of his sentence. What happened to the family from hereon is unknown and Bridget disappears from the records. John however, died of senility at the New Town Charitable Institution on 8 October 1894, age 75.

5 ♥ MARY ANN HALDANE

Although she cried bitterly when sentence was pronounced against her, Mary Ann was lucky to be arrested for housebreaking and sentenced to fourteen years transportation in November 1827. Had she not been, she may have faced the same fate as her mother and her sister. The notorious Burke and Hare in Edinburgh murdered both of them.

Seventeen-year-old Mary Ann had stolen from the house of Dr Thatcher of Eldon Street, Edinburgh. This was not her first offence. Born in Glasgow, Mary Ann moved to Edinburgh as a child. Her mother, Betty Haldane, lived at Westport and was a spinner, but Mary Ann lived apart from her mother at Castlebank where she was employed hawking eggs.

She had few skills and fewer opportunities, but she did have a friend, Margaret Finlayson, with whom she committed offences. The girls took their chances and helped each other out as they survived life on the city streets. At Mary Ann's trial one of the police officers reported that the girls were great companions, constantly walking about together and both very bad characters. Margaret, charged with theft in July 1827, was also sentenced to fourteen years and both she and Mary Ann were sent to London to sail to Van Diemen's Land together aboard the *Borneo* along with 71 other women. On arrival in Hobart Town in October 1828, the two girls were sent to properties outside Hobart Town. However, they were many miles apart. Mary Ann was in the Derwent Valley and Margaret was at Mona Vale near Ross. Margaret's record in the colony was clean, without colonial convictions. However Mary Ann was not so well behaved.

Back in Edinburgh, Irish immigrants William Burke and William Hare, along with Burke's de-facto, Helen McDougal, and Hare's wife, Margaret, hatched a plan to make some money by providing cadavers to Dr Robert Knox who lectured in anatomy at the Edinburgh Medical College. Paying up to £8 for each body used for dissection, Burke and Hare supplied up to sixteen corpses to Dr Knox, many of them they had murdered.

Mary Ann's mother, Betty, had fallen on hard times and in the spring of 1828 she asked if she could stay in Hare's house in Tanner's Close. Being partial to a drop of alcohol, one night, while sleeping off the effects of the night's drinks in the stable, Burke and Hare smothered her. Eventually Betty's daughter, Peggy or Margaret, came looking for her and she faced the same fate. The sensational story of the Burke and Hare murders was reported widely and Mary Ann may have learnt of the gruesome deaths of her sister and mother from the press.

While in the service of Mr McPherson Mary Ann gave birth. She was sent back to the House of Correction in January 1830 'being incumbered with a young child which she has had in her master's service'. Once Mary Ann weaned the child, she served her time in the Crime Class. In May 1831 at St Matthew's Church in New Norfolk, she married John Auton, a fellow convict also assigned to McPherson. It is likely that John was the father of her child. Two sons were born to the couple, John in 1832 and James in 1833. At the time the family was residing in the south of the colony. Mary Ann was assigned in the Swanport region in 1835 and at New Norfolk in 1836. She was returned to the Cascades Factory in June 1835, for disobedience of orders while assigned to her husband. A few months later, she spent fourteen days in solitary confinement on bread and water having been charged by Horton with over staying her pass. (Perhaps Horton was a misspelling of Auton or Horton was her master.)

Mary Ann's daughter Mary Ann Auton died as the result of a fire in a hut at Pittwater in May of 1839. She was probably the child whose birth led to Mary Ann's incarceration at the Cascades Female Factory in 1830. After this loss no offences were recorded until December 1839 when she was out after hours in 'the paddock', a notorious drinking and carousing spot at the time, and today known as the Domain in Hobart.

In March 1841 Mary Ann returned to Cascades for six months and her Ticket of Leave was suspended for drinking in a public house. John Auton was also charged with drinking in March 1841, and fined 5 shillings. By 1841 the Auton family was living back in Hobart where Mary Ann was again charged with misconduct and returned to the Factory to serve four months hard labour. She gained her Certificate of Freedom in November 1841 and her husband gained another Ticket of Leave in March 1841. John took up ploughing and advertised his services in the *Colonial Times*.

The family moved to Bridgewater and John and his two sons, John and James, became limeburners, burning limestone to make lime, a much needed product for building. John Auton junior died of inflammation, aged 21 at New Norfolk in July 1854. Tragedy struck again in September 1858 when John Auton senior, aged 68, died a horrendous and lingering death when his clothing caught fire in the taproom of the Bridgewater Hotel. James Auton married Louisa Marvell in 1860 at St John's New Town.

Mary Ann, aged 51, married a second time in February 1861. Her husband, John Cushion, was 58 and a former convict, and she had known him a while as he had witnessed James's marriage to Louisa. John Cushion died in 1879 at the New Town Pauper Establishment and from then on Mary Ann appeared to spend time in and out of the Charitable Institutions. She was discharged in November 1881, aged 70, as 'Able to Work'. After this, she disappears from the records. She outlived her mother and sister, two husbands, and two children. Two were murdered, two died as the result of fire. We can only hope that Mary Ann gained some joy from her numerous grandchildren born in the Bridgewater district. Many of their descendants today can tell the tale of Mary Ann Haldane, a survivor.

SARAH
MASON

♥ 6

Aged 21 when she arrived in Van Diemen's Land on board the *Aurora* (2) on 10 August 1851, Sarah Mason had been convicted of larceny, having stolen a shawl and a pair of boots from Mr Hancock of Manchester. Twice convicted before, Sarah was tried this time at the Manchester Borough Quarter Sessions and sentenced to seven years. Sarah was a house maid, single, Protestant and could read but not write. Her description on her record makes it sound as if there was little about Sarah's appearance that stood out—she had a medium sized head and forehead, medium sized nose, mouth and chin and no distinguishing marks.

One thing that is evident is that the most prominent feature of young Sarah was her determination and personality! Just six weeks after arriving, Sarah received her first introduction to the Cascades Female Factory for refusing to work while at the Brickfields Hiring Depot. Her sentence was fourteen days in the cells. When her fourteen days were over, Sarah returned to the Brickfields and moved between there and various employers in Hobart and New Town for the rest of the year.

On 26 January 1852 she absconded from the employ of G. Yeoland and was found to have committed 'larceny under the value of £5'. Her sentence was twelve months hard labour at the Cascades Female Factory. During the next twelve months Sarah found a myriad of ways to breach the rules and thus wound up with a total of nine days in solitary confinement, a week banned from exercise, almost a months worth of bread and water diet and considerable time at the wash tub.

Sarah's choices had landed her in the Female Factory just as the new regulations for houses of correction had been approved by J.S. Hampton, Comptroller General.

Every adult prisoner received into the Female House of Correction, Cascade, under a sentence of hard labour, shall be subjected to separate treatment for the first half of the period of her sentence ...

Each apartment will be furnished with a closely covered urinal, proper bedding, mess utensils and a Bible and Prayer Book, according to the religious persuasion of the occupant ...

The prisoners are strictly prohibited from holding any communication either by words or signs whilst in their apartment, at exercise, or in proceeding thereto or returning therefrom. They are positively forbidden to sing, read aloud or make any other noise in their apartment.

Sarah breached the 'silence' component of the regulations twice in her first six weeks in the Factory, once talking and the other for singing in her apartment. She managed to take the duty of a watchwoman without permission and three times received punishment for improper or disorderly conduct. Giving a piece of tobacco and leaving the yard without permission rounded out Sarah's entries in the Punishment book for 1852.

With her year of hard labour extinguished, on 2 December 1852 Sarah was assigned to T.Brown of Collins Street, Hobart, a position obviously not to Sarah's liking as by 4 December she had absconded. By January she was back in the Factory. For absconding she received an additional twelve months hard labour onto her sentence, this meant all of 1853 was to be spent within the walls of the Factory. It appears that Sarah toed the line until September when her offence was recorded as 'refusing to

have her hair cut' and received three days in solitary and a month back in the separate apartments.

Out two days after Christmas in 1853 and assigned to Mr Alberto of Bothwell, it seems that Sarah preferred the factory life, absconding again and returned to the Cascades for another eighteen months from January 1854. By mid-1855 she was posted to Snake Banks and was absent all night from her accommodation, being returned to the Factory for three months. The same thing happened when she was assigned to her next position—Sarah was out after hours and sent back to the Factory for ten days in solitary. Mr Dean of New Norfolk was her last listed assignment in March 1856, her Ticket of Leave being granted in September that same year.

On 4 November 1856 Sarah's application to marry James Sydenham was approved and twenty days later they were married in St. Mary the Virgin Church of England in Macquarie Plains. James was listed as a carpenter, and the couple presumably moved to the area in which they were married. The Police Office report for Hamilton from 31 December 1856, as reported in the *Hobarton Mercury* on 5 January 1857, recounts a brutal assault on James and Sarah by a man named

James Scully. James was charged with attacking the couple along with a man named James Dunn who had endeavoured to assist them. The report stated that they were 'much cut about their faces'. Scully was offered a fine of £5 or one month imprisonment with hard labour.

What happened to Sarah next is not known, but a woman of the same name and with the same year of birth passed away in Hobart on 21 January 1873, aged 43. James died a pauper in New Norfolk of disease of the heart and lungs in March 1890, at the age of 80.

MARY
DEVIGN

Convicted at the Surrey Assizes and sentenced to Death (commuted to transportation), Mary Devign was a highway robber. Her gaol report stated 'Bad character, connexions and disposition' and recorded that Mary was married with one child. In her statement, Mary named her husband as Robert Burke of the 57th Regiment and said her son was five years of age and lived in Lochrea, County Galway. Mary was an illiterate laundry maid, originally from Galway, and was 23 years of age when the *Mermaid* docked in Hobart on 27 June 1828.

The journey from Woolwich to Van Diemen's Land had not been easy on Mary, seeing her admitted on the sick list twice on board, in the first instance with 'hysteria'. Surgeon James Gilchrist's report went on to say:

Pretty orderly. 10 February 1828: Admitted on the sick-list with 'Hysteria': Has apparently been much dejected since she came on board. On the first evening (Tuesday 5th) she was suddenly seized with a paroxysm resembling Hysteria which was relieved by administering an Antispasmodea draught; this evening she had a similar attack, sudden, and attended with more violent spasms than the former ... States that she has been subject to these attacks for the last eight years, which at times have lasted for days without interruption. Her health in other respects is pretty good. Discharged cured, 15 February 1828. March 1828: Again admitted on the sick-list: Her complaints from the commencement have been decidedly of an hysterical nature and no doubt have been much aggravated by mental anxiety and irritation. Her character and conduct hitherto has been good tho' she possesses a violent temper when excited.

It is possible that Mary's bad temper and sudden violent spasms may today be diagnosed as something very different to hysteria?

Mary was a brunette with a fresh and freckled complexion, a small round head, sharp pointed nose, small and wrinkled forehead with a narrow temple. Her chin small, pointed and indented, her mouth was wide with large lips, she had grey eyes, a pockmark near the corner of her right eye and her eyebrows were 'thin of hair' and 'wide apart'. In the absence of a mug shot, Mary's detailed description may have come in handy on more than one occasion as she had a habit of absenting herself from work.

Ten of twenty colonial offences listed on her conduct record relate to neglecting her duties, being absent without leave or absconding. However, her first offence was nothing of the sort—it was fighting and creating a disturbance in the Factory just six weeks after arriving. For this, Mary received three days on bread and water in a cell. Perhaps she just wasn't any good at taking orders, as on numerous occasions during the five years of toing and froing between service and the Factory, Mary's refusal to follow directions shines through on her record.

The record of 20 February 1829 reads: 'Neglect of duty and being quite unserviceable to her Mistress'. On 23 March 1830 it is reported: 'Repeatedly absconding from her Master's service and refusing to obey his orders'. For this refusal to toe the line Mary was returned to the Factory for six months in Crime Class and to have her hair cut off. On 14 January 1831—'Neglect of duty in her service and absenting herself under false pretences'. It was back to the Factory. When assigned to Mr Davidson in July 1831, Mary was 'absent from her service the whole of last night without leave' and again was returned to the Factory, although interestingly 'Mr Davidson stating in every other respect she is a very hard working good servant'. It would appear that twelve months on, Mary's new employer did not agree with Mr Davidson as she was returned to Crime Class in the Factory for 'Neglecting her Mistress's Child & found in an indecent position on a bench in her Masters house'.

Between 1832 and 1835 Mary's refusal to work continued, as did a tendency to have one too many to drink, with a number of charges of being drunk and disorderly appearing on her conduct record. During this time Mary had two applications to marry rejected, one to Abel Hicken and the other to John Jelly. Third time lucky, her application to marry William Durham was approved on 16 January 1836. William, also a convict, was transported for 'machine breaking', and sentenced to seven years, but received his pardon just 21 days before the couple were wed on 24 February 1836 in Launceston. They were both in their fifties.

On 8 December 1837 Mary received her Ticket of Leave and on

17 March 1840, her Conditional Pardon. Where Mary and William went after receiving their respective freedoms is unknown.

SARAH
JACOBS

The Ratcliffe Highway in London's East End was a wild place, said a contemporary, 'headquarters of unbridled vice and drunken violence'. Its pubs were full of sailors on the summer's night in 1827 when Sarah Jacobs stole twenty sovereigns and eight £5 bank notes from John Thompson, who had just been paid by the Navy Office at Somerset House, and was waving his money around at the Ship and Shears. This was Sarah's territory, her beat as a 19-year-old prostitute, and the neighbourhood where she had been born and had lived all her life. The theft, followed by her arrest, trial and conviction at the Old Bailey, would separate her forever from the London docks, but it made no radical change in the way she lived.

In contrast to most convict women, Sarah continued to steal in Van Diemen's Land, though not immediately upon arrival on the *Mermaid*

in June 1828. The first five charges on her extensive conduct record were for disobeying orders, being insolent, getting drunk, and spending nights away from the houses of her (multiple) masters. Then, in October 1831, she was tried at the Hobart Town Quarter Sessions on a charge of stealing sixteen yards of lace from a shop. Surprisingly, and to Sarah's credit, her mistress 'gave her a good character for honesty and sobriety during a period of nearly a year'. Only six months before, a charge by the same mistress that Sarah had been drunk and disorderly had sent her out to the Cascades Female Factory for a week in a solitary cell on bread and water. After that episode, her mistress wanted her back, but theft of course was more serious. Sarah pleaded guilty, had another three years added to her fourteen year sentence—and apparently was not taken back.

From here on, no one seemed to speak up on Sarah's behalf and no one gave her a good character. The series of charges and punishments continued year after year as she shifted from master to master. In 1833 she was sent north to be assigned in the Launceston district and the next year was returned to the Launceston Female

Factory, being 'pregnant and unfit for service', but what happened to the pregnancy goes unrecorded. The next year she was charged on 'suspicion of felony' (probably another theft) but the charge does not stick. In 1837 a charge of larceny under £5 was proved, and her sentence extended another two years. She was sent south again, and spends as much time inside the Cascades Female Factory as out on assignment.

On 4 May 1839 Sarah was in the Crime Class when a riot broke out, an event brought to public attention by an unnamed newspaper 'correspondent' who wrote an account of prisoners in 'open rebellion' because they were given bread made from peas and barley instead of wheat. Sarah was among the 200 women who created a ferocious racket, broke the spinning wheels, 'armed themselves with the iron spindles' and large stones, and threatened to burn down the entire Factory. Fire engines raced out from Hobart Town. Meanwhile, a contingent of police arrived and broke down barricades erected by the prisoners. 'The rebellion', wrote the 'correspondent, 'was quelled,—and the building restored to Her Majesty'. And the prisoners, of course, were punished. Sarah was charged with 'insubordination ... in forcibly, violently and in a turbulent manner resisting Mr Hutchinson [the Superintendent] and with openly refusing to obey his lawful commands'. Her punishment was three months in the separate working cells and hard labour.

Sarah had now been under sentence in the colony for more than ten years, and she seems to have been completely alienated from the system of reform. Within weeks of her release from confinement in the separate working cells, she had been assigned to yet another master, had absconded, was facing another extension of a year on her sentence—and was back in the Female Factory for four months in the Crime Class. No sooner had she finished that punishment and been assigned than she was charged with theft of a chemise, received another extension of a year, and was back in the Crime Class again.

Finally, in April 1845, Sarah was granted a Ticket of Leave. Her next two charges were for the 'misconduct' of 'being in bed with a man'—punished in each case by two months hard labour inside the Female Factory. Who made the discovery? Was the real charge that she was living with a man? Perhaps Daniel Newman, who on 6 April 1846 applied to marry her. Approval was granted but there is no record of a marriage, or of what happened to Sarah after this. After so many years spent bucking the convict system, one wonders how Sarah could have settled into the routines of a normal family life or of community. When she arrived in Hobart, she identified herself as Jewish, one of a small group of women to do so, but there is no indication that she became involved in the local Jewish community who had banded together to build their synagogue. Sarah Jacobs had spent so many years on the move, it is hard to imagine her settling down. As far as the records show, she was free at the time of the convict muster in 1849, and after that she forever eludes the record-keepers.

NAPPY
RIBBON

The Great Famine of the late 1840s had taken its toll on the Irish population, and for women many were forced to crime. Animal theft was a common offence in the rural counties and in Galway, a 27-year-old country servant with the quirky name of Nappy Ribbon was tried before the courts on 23 June 1848 for stealing a sheep from Michael Joyce. She had previously been discharged by proclamation for the same offence, as Irish courts appeared reluctant to transport women for their first offence unless of a serious nature.

Nappy (a short form of Penelope) was married at the time. Her husband Patrick, along with her family consisting of father Michael, mother Kate, brothers Thomas, Patrick, John,

Michael, and William, and sisters Biddy, Catherine, and Bridget all resided in their native County Galway. She was of the Roman Catholic faith, illiterate and described as having a dark complexion, black hair, blue eyes, a round dimpled chin and a round scar on her forehead.

The minimum transportation sentence of seven years was Nappy's fate and within four months of her trial she found herself aboard the *Lord Auckland* (3) in Dublin with 200 female convicts bound for Van Diemen's Land. Departing in the early days of an Irish autumn, all but one of the women survived the 101 day voyage, arriving to a Hobart summer on 20 January 1849.

Assigned into service on arrival she conducted herself without offence until 27 May 1850 when, in Launceston, she refused to work for her master named Perrin. For this she was sentenced to ten days in the cells at the Launceston Female Factory. The father is unknown but quite possibly while in the service of Perrin, Nappy became pregnant. She gave birth to a son Thomas at the Female House of Correction in Launceston on 5 January 1851. By April 1852 she was assigned to Richard Davis in Launceston and on 6 July of that year received her Ticket of Leave and the opportunity to earn wages. No further reference to her son Thomas has been found—though with mortality rates high at the Female House of Correction, he may not have survived.

Meanwhile William Connor, a fellow convict, had also been assigned to Richard Davis three months before Nappy arrived. Transported to Norfolk Island aboard the *John Calvin* in 1846 for Life, he was then removed to Van Diemen's Land in 1847 to serve the remainder of his sentence. Though William relocated to W. Cogdell in Launceston on 19 August 1852, two days later, and four months after making her acquaintance, he and Nappy applied for permission to marry. No approval was forthcoming, and William remained with Cogdell until January 1853 when he transferred his service to Thomas Frost of Launceston.

Things came unstuck when on 19 October 1853 William and Nappy were brought before the magistrate in Launceston for living in adultery. Nappy was a Ticket of Leave holder at the time, and William claimed the same status, his previous applications for a Ticket having been refused. He received a sentence of six months hard labour at the Depot in Launceston, while Nappy was handed a four month sentence to hard labour at the Female House of Correction. She lost the indulgence of a Ticket of Leave, and appears to have lost touch with William. Despite this she may have given birth to his child when on 13 March 1854 Mary Ann Ribbon was born at the Launceston Female Factory. William stayed in the north of the colony around Launceston and Westbury, eventually gaining a Conditional Pardon in 1857.

After Mary Ann's birth, Nappy relocated to the Female Factory at Ross in June 1854, some five months before the institution was to close. Women might be here prior to assignment in the district, as well as under sentence, or accommodated because they had young infants as in Nappy's case. One of the reasons for its establishment had been to improve the environment for infants born to convict mothers, as mortality rates at the Hobart and Launceston Female Factories reflected badly on conditions there. However, any improvements to enhance the health of infants were unfortunately not to benefit young Mary Ann. On 10 July 1854 when at Campbell Town, Superintendent Dr George Everett confirmed her death of *catarrhus* (inflammation of mucous membranes, especially of the nose and throat)—she was only four months old.

With the closure of the Ross Female Factory, Nappy was relocated to the Female House of Correction at Cascades in Hobart prior to being assigned. One month after arriving at the household of Mrs Craven in Bathurst Street in February 1855, she was charged with insolence to her mistress. A kindly Mrs Craven, stating that Nappy was quite sober but very abusive, did not wish for her to be punished but also requested that she not return as her servant. The House of Correction was her only recourse before being assigned for a final time in April to Harvey in Elizabeth Street.

Two months later, on 26 June 1855, Nappy's sentence of transportation had expired and she gained her Free Certificate. Her behaviour following her arrival reflected that of many other Irish men and women transported during the time of the famine. Many were first offenders and were relatively well behaved following their arrival. Nappy had only committed three seemingly minor offences between 1849 and 1855.

The last reference found to Nappy Ribbon is on 8 July 1858 when, at the age of 33, she married Joseph Harvey at the house of William Pow in the River Leven District of Port Sorell. Married according to the rites and ceremonies of the Independent Church by the Reverend Walter Mathison she was listed as a widow and servant, Joseph as a labourer. They appear to have had no children, and their subsequent life is a mystery, though a notice in the *Launceston Examiner* in June and July 1870 may link to

an ensuing life on the land—if they had stayed in the River Leven district: *July 8th [1870]. E.F. Dease is instructed to sell by auction on the premises on Friday 8th July, at one o'clock, the whole of the stock and other goods of Joseph Harvey, farmer, River Leven – 2 good plough and cart mares, 1 foal – first class, 2 cows, 2 heifers, 3 yearlings, 15 pigs, 2 bags seed wheat, 7 bags seed oats, 7 bushels rye grass seed, 5 bags flour, 1 plough, 1 pair harrows, 2 sets plough harness, 1 cart saddle, 1 saddle and bridle, 1 cross-cut saw, maul and wedges, quantity tools, fowls, wheat, etc. etc. Terms cash. No reserve.*

MARY MCLAUCHLAN

As a local newspaper reminded its readers, the hanging of Mary McLauchlan on 19 April 1830 marked 'the first instance of a woman being brought to the scaffold in Van Diemen's Land'. Her execution is brutally evident, and yet the events leading up to it remain hauntingly elusive.

When Mary was arrested in Glasgow early in November 1827, she said that 'she is 23 years of age, is wife of William Sutherland, weaver', and 'is overseer of ten girls employed in picking cotton in William Dunlop's Mill'. This was Mary's first arrest. 'Connexions respectable' said her gaol report, 'and former course of life good'. So why did she steal every piece of clothing, bedding, and linen belonging to a woman she knew? Money was not the motive, because she neither sold nor pawned the stolen goods, but simply stored them in a coal cellar. No one suspected Mary until she brazenly wore one of the stolen caps when she went to visit a neighbour who was, as she well knew, the victim's closest friend. 'Look at me', she seemed to say. And of course they all did. She was still wearing that cap when the policeman came to her house and took the evidence of theft from her head.

A year later Mary was sailing on the *Harmony,* a prisoner sentenced to fourteen years transportation. Two years later she was in the Crime Class of the Cascades Female Factory, and pregnant.

In January 1829 when the *Harmony* disembarked its human cargo on the wharf of Hobart Town, Mary was assigned to a settler farming in the Coal River Valley, Charles Ross Nairne. She remained at 'Glen Nairne' for seven months, and then her master charged her with 'misconduct'. Mary responded with a counter charge, 'stating she has not received the proper quantity of clothing'. The Principal Superintendent of Convicts took this charge seriously, and ordered her to the Female Factory until Mrs Nairne could be brought into town to answer.

And then, after this decision, something happened to make the Principal Superintendent radically change his mind, and come down hard on Mary for 'making a charge against her Master and Mistress which when investigated is found to be without any foundation'. For this false accusation she was to be punished severely—six days in a cell on bread and water, six months in the Crime Class, then assignment in the Interior.

The next recorded mention of Mary McLauchlan comes almost eight months later when three newspapers report her sensational trial, a subject of gossip throughout the colony. At a time when newspapers routinely devoted column after column to verbatim reporting, they shied away from this newsworthy story. The longest account is a stark summary in the *Colonial Times:*

Mary MacLachlan [sic], was placed at the bar charged with the wilful murder of her new born male child, it appeared that the prisoner had been privately delivered of a child whilst confined in the female house of correction, and had caused its death by strangulation and afterwards concealed it in the water closet. A vast number of witnesses, were examined and after a most [sic] and patient investigation, lasting from the morning until late in the evening, the prisoner, was found Guilty, and sentenced to be executed on Saturday morning, and her body to be dissected. This is only the second instance of a female being tried for murder, in this Colony and the first convicted of the offence.

What was going on? How could a prisoner in the communal space of the Crime Class at Cascades be 'privately delivered of a child'? Even the privies (water closets) were not 'private', and certainly not a reflection of the individual cubicles in today's toilet blocks that we are all used to. Why wasn't Mary in the institution's hospital? Should not the Lovells, as Superintendent and Matron, have monitored the heavily pregnant prisoner? After all, the new Female Factory—barely a year old—had not yet become the overcrowded space of later years.

Inside the prison there was no secret hiding place, nothing like the coal cellar in Glasgow. The privy might hide a baby's body for a brief moment, but it was an obvious place for a search. And a search was inevitable if a woman was heavily pregnant one day and not the next.

Putting the body in the privy was rather like wearing the stolen cap. It called attention to a crime. At a stage in medical history when it was notoriously difficult to decide whether a baby had been born dead (strangled perhaps with the cord around its neck), or smothered at birth, Mary might simply have handed over the dead child, and claimed it was stillborn. Concealing the body triggered a scenario of foul play. Now there would have to be an inquest, which probably took place inside the Female Factory. But why the inquest's verdict of 'wilful murder', a verdict in no-one's interest, revealing a breakdown in surveillance inside this brand new institution?

Even after the 'vast number of witnesses' gave their evidence in the day-long public trial, disturbing questions remained. Mary was reprieved for the weekend to give Lieutenant-Governor Arthur time to take advice from his Executive Council. All Saturday afternoon they met, and again on Sunday. Though they were not unanimous, they did not recommend mercy.

On Monday morning Mary McLauchlan ascended the gallows. She wore a white dress tied at the waist with a black ribbon. As she had promised the attending clergyman, she did not reveal to onlookers the name of her baby's father (rumoured to be her master Charles Nairne) and exclaimed only 'Oh, my God!' as she fell.

Mary McLauchlan is a troubling figure, a victim no doubt of a colonial justice system that withheld the mercy often extended in Britain to mothers accused of infanticide. And yet there may have been something about Mary that did not invite mercy, some disturbing behavioural trait that alienated the very people who might have helped her. With no surviving records of the inquest or of witness statements at her trial, with no account from Mary herself, we are left wondering who she really was and what happened when she gave birth inside the Female Factory.

MARY
WILKES

Things did not start well in Van Diemen's Land for Mary Wilkes. Before she had set foot in the colony, she was in trouble. Mary's conduct on the voyage was quarrelsome, defiant and disorderly and she tried to encourage others to follow her example. The surgeon on the *Sovereign*, Robert Malcolm, was not impressed and nor was the magistrate who sent her straight to the Factory once she disembarked. For her misdemeanours, Mary was to spend fourteen days on bread and water in a cell at the Hobart Town Female Factory.

Mary was just 22, a girl from Bromyard in Herefordshire, when she was charged with highway robbery at the Warwick Assizes in March 1827. She was a hawker, but said she could also cook a plain dinner, wash and iron. When she first set foot in Hobart Town, she probably stepped onto a small jetty on what had been Hunter's Island. From there she would have walked up Macquarie Street past the Hobart Town rivulet, Government House, the Commissariat Stores, the Courthouse and St David's Church. At the corner of Murray Street, she would have been marched into the old gaol. From the gaol, Mary went into service under the Assignment System. This meant that Mary was not paid for her toil and that she could be returned at any time should her employer find her behaviour unsatisfactory. Her master had to provide Mary with clothing, bedding and rations. If she was ill, he was to provide medical treatment.

Working at the Crown Inn on the Coal River Road was probably not a sensible place to assign a girl with a liking for drink. Drink got Mary into trouble and in July 1828 she was back in a cell for seven days. Mary was repeatedly absent from her work and repeatedly drunk. Her next master was William Abel Jnr who lived in the Macquarie District. William was the son of an ex-convict and publican who for a time ran the Kings Head Inn at New Norfolk. Drink got the better of Mary again and this time she spent a week in the solitary cells at the new Cascades Factory. Mary returned to work for Abel, but six months later she absconded. However, she did not go alone.

Edward Taylor, a gardener from Lincolnshire was charged with enticing Mary Wilkes, a runaway convict, to live in the bush with him. How they survived for five months in the Tasmanian bush in the autumn and early winter of 1829 remains a mystery. From her trial records, we know that Mary disguised herself by wearing men's clothing. Was this for warmth, for protection, or just a convenient disguise? Once discovered, Mary and Edward faced the magistrate on 11 June 1829. Edward was to work in irons for two years. Mary was sent to Cascades for a year. It is surprising that she was again charged with absconding in the September of the same year. In fact, she ran away from a Constable who had her in his charge and she got drunk again. She was back in the Crime Class in a cell for ten days on bread and water.

Mary left Abel's employment and in 1830 was charged three times for drunkenness and refusing to go to the House of Correction. At this time she was in the employ of Mr Harper. In early 1832 Mary assaulted her then master, Mr Broad. After two months in Cascades she did not return to his service, but instead was assigned to Lieutenant Carter and to Mr Nairne. After being charged with drunkenness four times during that year, Mr Nairne not unsurprisingly returned her to the service of the Crown. Apparently two stints in the solitary cells had not dampened her taste for liquor. In 1832 she absconded another three times. Once she got as far as Launceston and was free of servitude for almost a month. On one occasion she handed herself in after a month at large and on another she absconded from the constable while being taken back to the Factory. Penal servitude did not suit Mary.

In 1834 Mary was at Ross working for Thomas Anstey, a retired police magistrate, at his property 'Anstey Park' near Oatlands. She probably worked in the house known as Anstey Barton. Her behaviour was not to Anstey's liking. Mary was frequently intoxicated, swore profanely, her behaviour was violent and outrageous and she resisted the constable sent to remove her. After six months in the Factory, she did not return to the Anstey property. This was Mary's last recorded incarceration in Cascades. She had been one of the first women locked in the new solitary cells and had spent about four months locked in those cells because of her 19 offences. She was no stranger to hard labour or the Crime Class.

It took Mary a long time to gain any indulgence. Because she was transported for Life, she had to serve eight years before she could apply for a Ticket of Leave and in 1836 she was granted her Ticket. In November 1840 Mary's Conditional Pardon was approved. By this time, she was married to Mr J. Laurence as recorded at the time of the 1835 muster. The marriage registration has not been found, but there were several convicts of the name Laurence or Lawrence who may have partnered Mary. In 1842 she was mustered at Bothwell. Then Mary disappears from the public record. This was not unusual—many women reinvented themselves, moved, and changed their names. Sometimes they died forgotten, unregistered.

Did Mary ever tell stories of her survival in the bush? Certainly, she would have had tales to tell. She was no ordinary runaway convict.

MARY
KENNEDY

On 23 April 1865 Mary Ann Gardiner (formerly Kennedy) died of pleuro-pneumonia in the Hobart General Hospital. She was only 37.

Fourteen years earlier, Mary Kennedy had arrived in Hobart aboard the convict transport *Aurora* (2). Married at the time, a washerwoman and a native of Glasgow, she had previously faced a magistrate on three occasions—once for stealing, and twice for quarrelling. Her family included husband James, mother Catherine, and three sisters Biddy, Catherine and Rosannah. On 24 December 1850 she was brought before the Court of Justiciary in Glasgow for stealing a gown. Sentenced to seven years transportation, and described as 'very good' on board the voyage, she arrived in Van Diemen's Land at a time when transportation of convicts was coming to a close.

With the Probation System virtually ended, Mary, along with other female convicts who arrived from 1850, was assigned to domestic service on arrival. Within five days of landing in Hobart she was assigned to Mr W.C. Robertson of Hampden Road, Battery Point, but within six months she was to experience life at the Cascades Female Factory, having been found to be drunk when in Robertson's service. To what appears to be a harsh sentence of six months hard labour, she responded in coming months by being neglectful in her duty at the Factory and allowing talking in the ward after the silence bell had been rung.

Returning to assigned service, this time to Daniel O'Leary of Cascades, three months had barely passed before she was returned to the Female Factory again for being absent and drunk. This pattern of drunkenness was repeated on a number of occasions, and following form she was disorderly, neglectful and disobedient when returned to confinement.

Up until June 1853, Mary had spent her time in domestic service in Hobart, but then moved briefly to the Huon district before reoffending and being ordered not to again enter service in Hobart Town. From then on, between stints at the Female Factory, she was assigned to Jerusalem (now Colebrook), and then to Thomas Terry of the property 'Slateford', New Norfolk, for three months in September 1853. At the time, he had three children less than nine years of age—two others having died in recent years. Being a farming property, life would have been busy, and Mary's assistance to Thomas's wife Elizabeth would have been appreciated, but she was found drunk on three occasions during her time there. It is worth noting that just prior to her going to 'Slateford' she had applied in July and September for permission to marry Benjamin Baker, but

the application was refused. Many convicts on seven year sentences were permitted to marry after only three years. However, rules were relaxed at times, but for Mary only two years had passed when she applied. She would still have been regarded as 'married' to her husband in England, and her repeated drunkenness may also have influenced the decision as many such women were regularly denied the indulgence.

Mary gained a Ticket of Leave in May 1856, and it wasn't until December of that year that she applied for permission to marry again, this time to John Gardiner, listed as free, and approval was given. There is no evidence that John was ever a convict. They married at St George's Church in Hobart on 22 December 1856. John was a 23-year-old blacksmith.

Mary's further assignments had mostly been in the Hamilton district, and though now free to work for wages, being on a Ticket of Leave, she was brought before the magistrate on four occasions for drunkenness, obscene language and disturbing the peace. In most cases she was fined.

On 18 January 1858, at Fingal, the last offence noted on her conduct record was for falsely representing herself to be free, for which she received a sentence of four months hard labour. She returned to the Female Factory and in marked variance to her previous conduct there, she was well behaved. Though her 'home' after marrying John is not known, by the time she arrived at the Factory to serve her sentence she was pregnant, and in April 1858 gave birth to a daughter Mary. John is listed on the birth certificate as a labourer. Just prior to this, she received a remission of the unexpired portion of a sentence extension given in 1854 for a larceny offence, and in May 1858 Mary gained her Free Certificate.

Within seven years her life was cut short. Struck down by a combination of pleurisy and pneumonia, 'symptoms begin with chilliness and shivering ... followed by fever, thirst and restlessness and a violent pricking pain which ... is most great when the patient breathes in'. Autumn was in the air in Hobart but weather had been generally mild, not much wind, and little rain. These were generally conditions '... favourable to health and life', though temperatures on the night before Mary died dropped to three degrees Celsius and whatever had caused her ailing condition, she wasn't to survive, leaving behind a husband and seven-year-old daughter. Their fate is unknown.

ELIZABETH CATO

Elizabeth Burgess was born and baptised in Ticehurst, Sussex, England in September 1800 to parents Thomas, a labourer, and Elizabeth Burgess. Where and how Elizabeth met locksmith William Cato is unknown, but the couple were married at St Mary's in the parish of Lambeth, London on 26 September 1822. Nearly twelve months later, the couple had their first child, also named William. In the following year Elizabeth gave birth to a girl, Sophia. The couple's second son, Joseph, was born in August 1826, a son Edward in May of 1828 and finally a daughter Elizabeth in September 1829.

What it was that prompted the Catos to leave their homeland with the intention of joining the fledgling colony of the Swan River in Western Australia is a mystery, but they lined up to take passage on one of the three ships arranged by Thomas Peel transporting free settlers to his new settlement. Unfortunately for the Catos, it appears they took passage on the final ship, the *Rockingham*.

The *Rockingham* arrived off Garden Island on 12 May 1830 with 172 colonists on board. The vessel dropped anchor off Clarence, the settler camp on the mainland side of

Cockburn Sound. At the same time a violent storm hit and carried the boats with the first wave of disembarking passengers (the single men) straight to the mainland shore, overturning them in the surf.

The storm dragged the large ship broadside onto the beach hitting one of its quarter boats, which luckily was still able to be used to transport the remaining passengers (married men and their families) to shore. With the help of those who had already landed, most of the families reached the shore safely, only a few having to wade ashore.

It is believed that the passengers spent the night on the beach in poor weather until the ship could be accessed the following day. Many of the food stores and supplies had been inundated with salt water, and the livestock had swum ashore and dispersed. It is not surprising that the Catos appear to have taken the opportunity to join the mass exodus from the western colony bound for Van Diemen's Land. This movement is recorded in a letter in the publication *The Athenæum* in 1831:

Emigration to this highly favoured land (Van Diemen's Land) increases rapidly: nearly one hundred passengers have arrived from England during week, and nearly one hundred more are daily expected from Swan River. Reports brought by of the vessels that arrived lately say that place is about to be evacuated. When the Cleopatra *left the Swan River, the* Eagle *was loading for Hobart Town.*

Arriving in Hobart on board the schooner *Eagle* on 30 January 1831, the *Colonial Times* lists 'Mrs Cato and children' on the passenger list. Whether William came ahead or later is unclear, however they both accepted positions at the Cascades Female Factory in April 1831. The Catos took the roles of Assistant Superintendent and Assistant Matron.

The Factory itself was experiencing a major growth period and overcrowding was rife. When the Catos arrived a second yard was under construction, to alleviate congestion in the convict accommodation and the conditions. In particular the mortality within the walls of the Factory was under scrutiny in the local press. In early 1832 after the Hutchinsons arrived at the Factory as Superintendent and Matron, Lieutenant-Governor Arthur inspected the Factory himself amid reports of the unsavoury conditions. Arthur found bugs and fleas everywhere, describing the conditions as being the worst among the children, their bedding as 'quite black with fleas'.

During her ten years of employment at the Factory, Elizabeth saw many changes take place, including developments to combat crowding, a shift in punishment away from the iron collar and a new Governor to replace Arthur in Sir John Franklin. It must have been quite hard for Elizabeth to care for her children and be working assisting Matron Hutchinson in her considerable duties, managing hundreds of women on a daily basis. Yet time after time, despite efforts to improve the conditions within the walls, the establishment was under scrutiny from the world outside. After the investigation that resulted in the Hutchinson's predecessors leaving in 1831, another was initiated during Franklin's first year in office. Page five of the *Colonial Times* in March 1838 reports:

> The mismanagement of the Female House of Correction is, at last, likely to become invest-igated, as some discoveries have been made of a frightful and most disgusting nature. We have always considered, that great alteration was required both in the moral and physical manage-ment of this establishment.

The article goes on to criticise Mary Hutchinson for not performing her duties with 'that attention to impartiality and fairness', which ought to character-ise it. Page seven of the same issue surprisingly takes a different tack:

> There is the devil to pay about the Factory, and a clean sweep is expected to be the consequence. We hope, however, that whatever change may take place, the services of Mr. and Mrs. Cato may be still retained at that establishment. The extreme civility of the Assistant Superintend-ent and his wife are well known to all; and their kindness to some of the poor creatures, incarcerated in that gloomy cavern, has gained

> them many a blessing, even from the lips of the most reprobate.

It seems that both the press and the convicts noticed the difference in management styles between Elizabeth and Mary, and perhaps this was the case, or was it just playing the age-old roles of good cop, bad cop?

Reporting on a Jury visit to the Factory during late March 1838, the *Colonial Times* gave thanks to the Catos: 'We must not omit to mention the praise, which is due to Mr and Mrs Cato ... for the readiness with which they attend to all the enquiries of the Jury; as contrast to that of the Matron'.

It would appear that Elizabeth's kindness towards the prisoners would be the couple's undoing. The *Sydney Gazette* (17 April 1841) reported the story under the title 'A Specimen of Penal Discipline'. According to the article, a married woman confined within the establish-ment wrote a letter to her husband requesting that he send items prohib-ited under the Factory regulations addressed to Mrs Cato and send them with a fowl as inducement. The letter somehow made its way into the hand of Mr John Price (Police Magistrate). The Catos admitted to the occurrence of the wrong doing and were ordered to be dismissed by Governor Franklin. However he allowed them to stay in the roles until replacements were found later that year.

In 1842 Elizabeth and William were in Richmond where William became a carrier. On his passing in 1843, Elizabeth posted an advertisement thanking the public for their support and announcing that she was hoping to continue the business 'for the benefit of herself and family'. Less than twelve months after posting that ad, Elizabeth passed away, aged just 43 years of age. She was buried in St Luke's at Richmond.

SARAH
NEWALL

Sarah Newall was twenty years old when transported to the other side of the world for 'stealing money from a person'. The grand sum of 18 shillings her undoing, although she admitted having spent five months in prison for shoplifting and having been brought before the Sessions twice prior to her latest effort. Sentenced to seven years transportation, Sarah would leave behind her parents and three siblings.

Along with 231 other female convicts, 35 free adults and children, Sarah sailed from London in April 1851, bound for Van Diemen's Land. A housemaid from Manchester, her physical description suggests life

hadn't been easy. She bore a scar on her left cheek and one between her eyebrows, and at some stage she had been bled from her left arm. The bloodletting may have occurred as a result of the diagnosis of *ulcus anthrax* (a skin ulcer linked to anthrax) on board the *Aurora* (2) on 9 August 1851, just one day before the vessel docked in Hobart on 10 August. While the other 228 female convicts who survived the journey (3 died during the voyage) disembarked on their way to serve their sentences, Sarah was admitted directly to the Colonial Hospital.

After a few weeks she was released from hospital to the Brickfields Hiring Depot and immediately assigned. Her 'bad' character on board the ship didn't resurface until March 1852, when she was charged with absconding from her place of employment and sentenced to nine months hard labour at the Cascades Female Factory. While confined within the Factory walls, Sarah spent over 30 days in solitary for disorderly conduct when employed as a cook, being asleep on her post and absent without leave.

In March 1853 assignment to a household in Sandy Bay was not to her liking and she absconded from duty, again finding herself in the House of Correction, this time only in transit before being relocated to the Ross Female Factory. From February 1854 for the next ten months Sarah worked for a number of people in both Campbell Town and Ross.

It was most likely during her time in the midlands that she met John Warren, a coachman, and on 1 August 1854 Sarah made an application for permission to marry John. On 18 September 1854 they married in St Luke's Church, Campbell Town and life was looking up. Within eight weeks Sarah gained a Ticket of Leave and about a week later gave birth to a daughter, Mary Ann Warren.

Details of the next six years of Sarah and John's life together are sketchy. However, if you believe what you read in the newspapers, everything was not happily ever after. The *Cornwall Chronicle* reported on Saturday 16 March 1861 Sarah—along with five others—was charged with assaulting John with intent to do him grievous bodily harm. The assault took place in the couple's Tamar Street home, police finding John lying on the floor, undressed, in a pool of blood. At first the police believed John dead due to his insensibility, and as a result of his being unable to communicate who had attacked him all the residents of the three row cottages were taken into custody.

John was taken to the Cornwall Hospital and when he came around,

told police that there was no need to have everyone under arrest on his account as it was Sarah who assaulted him. The Police Magistrate gathered evidence from John on 25 March while he was still in hospital. On the night of the assault, Sarah had claimed she was out getting candles when John was assaulted—John's evidence was quite contradictory.

I am the husband of Sarah Warren, now present, I lately resided in Tamar Street. On the night of the 16th instant, my wife and I were there about ten o'clock, she was not sober and I had two or three glasses also ... She came into the bedroom and went to the safe to get some food for the child. Asked her if she was coming to bed, she replied she was not, and that she was going out again. Said she should not and caught hold of her. We struggled together, and in the struggle I was wounded in the nose, I believe by the knife she had in her hand. Bled very much. Do not know who assisted me or first came in; believe Hone was the first. There was no-one in the house but my wife and child when I was wounded. Do not know what statement I may have previously made, but what I say now is correct.

One of the five people originally arrested with Sarah was Mr Robert Hone, a neighbour to the Warrens. He gave the following evidence:

I had had a glass or two, but I was sober; I was going to bed about 10 o'clock when John Warren called out to me Bob, for God's sake come in I'm bleeding to death; … I took no notice, but said "go to sleep Jack"; then the prisoner called me … I went round and found the backdoor open; Warren was lying on the floor in the bed room with his head in a pool of blood. I asked the prisoner who done it three of four times. She gave me no answer, but was crying … I did not go into Warren's when he first called, because rows are frequent there when there is a drop of drink about.

With accusations flying, Sarah was held in remand until John was fit enough to be discharged from hospital and give another statement, although when he repeated his statement the Police Magistrate chose to drop the charges against Sarah.

Despite her 'disorderly' nature throughout the 1860s, she appears considerate of others. In 1876 Sarah observed 70-year-old Mr James Murrell wander into a water closet and take considerable time in there, on checking to see if he was okay she discovered he had hanged himself. It would be just four years later that Sarah would also meet her sad end.

Just after 2am on 14 February 1882 a fire broke out in Lower Tamar Street, Launceston, in a house belonging to Mr H. Clayfield. It was a quarter of an hour before the fire was discovered and by the time the fire brigade arrived, the house was completely destroyed. Neighbours had attempted to extinguish the fire to no avail and once the fire brigade had quelled the flames, a body was found amid the ruins, close to the fireplace near the sofa. As the body was 'charred out of all resemblance to a human form' the coroner and jury accorded an open verdict, despite statements from neighbours and Ann Young who had lived with Sarah for a while suggesting that the body resembled Sarah.

The whereabouts of John and their daughter Mary Ann during this awful event are unknown, although the *Examiner* reported on 16 February 'there is no doubt now as to the identity' and a few friends had subsidised the amount the government had paid to the undertaker to permit a 'very nice coffin' for Sarah. Perhaps those friends were her family?

ELIZABETH ROBERTS

For almost ten years Elizabeth Roberts' sentence to transportation looked like the ticket to a better life than the one left behind in Liverpool where she had been convicted of stealing coral beads. Elizabeth was a girl of sixteen when she arrived in Hobart Town on the *Garland Grove* (2) in January 1843, a memorable lass with red hair and light blue eyes.

Elizabeth accepted the routines of convict life, chalking up only three charges on her conduct record. Once in the Brickfields Hiring Depot she got into some sort of trouble about her cap and was carted across town to the Cascades Female Factory for three months hard labour. The next year she stood before a magistrate charged with insolence, but either the charge seemed petty or her side of the story believable because the case was dismissed.

After she had been in the colony for just two years of her ten-year sentence, Elizabeth was granted a Ticket of Leave, though she came close to losing it a little later when she was charged with being out after hours. Perhaps she had been enjoying the company of Michael Arkwright, who applied to marry her on 9 March 1846. Once the marriage was approved, the couple apparently considered themselves married without darkening the doors of a church. On 27 April 1846 the first of their four children was born, Mary Ann. Elizabeth Arkwright nee Roberts registered the birth, signing with an 'X'. In 1848 William Arkwright was born, followed in 1851 by John and in 1853 by Ellen.

These were the most stable and prosperous years of Elizabeth's adult life. Her husband was ambitious, and he was in the process of transform-

ing himself from convict into colonist. Where the money came from is unclear, though his name on shipping arrivals and departures (he travelled cabin class) suggests he may have done well from the goldrush.

Property was the key to improving status for convict emancipists, and it was as a 'householder' in the district of Hobart that Michael's name appeared on a list of electors published by the *Colonial Times* in September 1851. By the beginning of 1853 he was the licensee of the Cross Keys Hotel in Liverpool Street, and his name was often printed in the newspapers as one of the citizens (male) petitioning for this and that. Elizabeth was now in her late twenties, the mother of four children and wife of a publican. More than ten years had passed since her trial, she was free, and she had a future.

And then everything fell apart. Although Michael Arkwright bought the Royal Oak hotel in Watchorn Street from its licensed owner, a new Licensing Act made serving alcohol illegal until the official transfer of license on a government-designated 'Transfer Day'. To make this point, the police targeted the convict turned publican, and in January 1855 Michael was fined a hefty £20 for serving half a pint of ale. A couple of weeks later, the transfer became official. Within a fortnight, the police swooped again, this time charging Michael with Sunday trading. 'Guilty', your Honour, 'to having the door open to admit a lodger' said Michael. The sanctimonious judge 'observed, that Sunday trading, and night-drinking had so much increased, that he, for one, should be inclined to indict heavy penalties'. Continued fines and harassment drove Michael Arkwright out of business, and when the cutter in which he was part-owner was driven onto Sandy Bay Point during a gale, the convict emancipist had had enough. He left the colony.

The family fell apart. In March 1856 the three oldest Arkwright children were admitted to the Queen's Orphan Schools, followed in November by their little sister Ellen. Elizabeth Roberts was drinking and destitute, and yet giving up her children was terrible. In April 1857 she persuaded the Orphan School officials that she could now take proper care of Ellen, though it is hard to see why they believed her. In May 1858 mother and daughter were living in a right-of-way off the Old Wharf. Four year-old Ellen was on her own in the yard behind the Sailors Return when her clothes caught fire. Probably her screams alerted someone who found the badly burnt child and went for the doctor who sent her to the General Hospital, where she died in agony a fortnight later.

The next year Elizabeth retrieved her oldest daughter from the Orphan School, thinking perhaps that thirteen-year-old Mary Ann could find work to support her mother. If so, the arrangement didn't last long, and Mary Ann took off on her own. From now on, Elizabeth Roberts is visible only when she was hauled into the Police Court on a charge of disturbing the peace or brawling.

Elizabeth's sons spent their childhoods in the Orphan School, and were then apprenticed. William stayed throughout his apprenticeship with a single master in Sandy Bay, but John could not settle. He absconded from one master, stole a gun from another. Then, when he was seventeen, the stout-built lad with reddish hair inherited from his mother found himself imprisoned for a year in Hobart Gaol. The cycle of crime and punishment turned round again. In 1865 Elizabeth too was imprisoned once more, sentenced to a month of hard labour on yet another charge of using obscene language. All the hopefulness from the years when Michael was a publican and she was the mother of a family had drained away.

ANN CATCHLOVE

♣3

Nineteen-year-old Ann Catchlove was a nursery maid and needlewoman when she arrived in Van Diemen's Land on the convict ship *Anna Maria* (2) on 26 January 1852. Tried in Sussex at Horsham Assizes in July 1851, Ann was sentenced to transportation for fifteen years for larceny. It was not her first offence for theft—her gaol report stated that she was 'thrice convicted'. To add to this, she had been twelve months 'on the town'. Ann believed that she had been transported for receiving a watch.

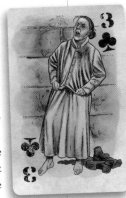

In 1851 Ann was living at home with her parents and four siblings in Westbourne, Sussex, where she was born. Her father was a chairmaker and Ann and two brothers were also chairmakers. There is no evidence that she used her chairmaking expertise in Van Diemen's Land, where her skills as a nursery maid and needlewoman were much more marketable.

As were all convicts at this time, Ann was interviewed when she arrived in Van Diemen's Land and her physical description and other details were recorded on her convict conduct record. Single and literate, she was described as having a fair complexion, dark brown hair, dark hazel eyes, and a small mouth, nose and chin.

Ann was unsettled almost from the time of her arrival. Initially she was assigned in Hobart with a brief spell at the New Town Farm in February 1852 and the following month at the Brickfields. She was in the colony just over a month when she absconded. From April 1852 Ann was in the Cascades Female Factory, where she was ordered to undergo twelve months probation. While there, in July 1852, she was allocated employment suitable to her needlework skills—making up curtains—but even this got her into trouble. She could not 'satisfactorily account' for the materials and was sentenced to four months hard labour. On top of this, she was accused of disrespectful conduct and was sentenced to fourteen days hard labour.

In August 1852, still in the Factory, Ann was sentenced to fourteen days in the cells for disorderly conduct in the work room. In September that year, she was charged with singing and making a noise in her cell and was punished with ten days in the cells.

Just after the start of the New Year in 1853, the reason for Ann's erratic behaviour became apparent. Still at the Cascades Female Factory, she was admitted to the Asylum for the Insane at New Norfolk. Her case notes recorded that she was subject to 'periodical attacks of insanity, combined to some extent with Hysteria'—she was noisy, abusive and violent. The notes added that she was an English girl, unmarried and only twelve months in the colony. Although she could read and write, her health had never been good and she 'always suffered from her head'. Her head was shaved three times before she left England.

Ann suffered from an irritable temper and she stated that 'her habits have not been intemperate—she dare not drink as a very little affects her head'. Her mother was in a lunatic asylum near London. Ann was still in the Asylum at New Norfolk in May 1853 when, in an excited state, she struck one of the nurses. By December, she had recovered—her health was good and she was free from headache. Quiet, well-behaved and very industrious, Ann appeared rational and coherent and was considered fit for discharge.

A month after leaving the Asylum, Ann's marriage to fellow convict Samuel Layton was approved. In February 1854 they married in St Matthew's Church of England at New Norfolk. Samuel, who arrived on the *Rodney* (2) in December 1851, had been convicted of sheep stealing in England in 1848 and was sentenced to transportation for ten years. Well behaved in the colony, he was granted a Conditional Pardon in July 1854.

Ann and Samuel, who were living in Argyle Street, had a daughter in Hobart in October 1854. At the time of the child's birth, Samuel was a farrier (he had been a groom and colt-breaker in England). Ann registered the birth, signing her mark 'X'—despite having been previously recorded as literate. The child, Angelina Layton, died of 'debility' (feebleness) on 6 January 1855. No further children have been located.

Ann was granted a Ticket of Leave in April 1855 and was recommended for a Conditional Pardon in January 1856, which was approved in November 1856. No record of her has been located after this date.

Ann's husband, Samuel Layton, may have left the colony for Sydney in November 1855.

BRIDGET MURPHY

Bridget Murphy, a country servant from Kerry, departed Dublin on 22 November 1846 on the *Arabian* and arrived in Hobart at the end of February 1847. Previously imprisoned for three months for stealing a shawl, she was tried in Kerry in June 1846 and transported for seven years for stealing a cloak. Although well-behaved in gaol, her behaviour during the voyage was recorded by the surgeon as 'bad'. While no detail was provided, it was perhaps a sign of the turbulence to come.

At twenty Bridget was leaving behind in Ireland her father, two brothers and a sister. Roman Catholic, illiterate and single, she was 5 feet 5 inches tall with a fresh complexion, black hair and hazel eyes. She had a large sharp nose, large mouth and sharp chin, and kept her mouth half open. She had tattoos on both hands, a blue ring on each middle finger.

On arrival in Hobart, Bridget was placed on the hulk *Anson* in the River Derwent—it kept the new arrivals separate from the old hands and also provided a location for training in domestic service. While on the *Anson*, in April 1847, Bridget was charged with misconduct for having two loaves of bread in her possession. As punishment her existing term of probation was extended three months. The usual period on the *Anson* was six months but Bridget was still there in February 1848, when she was sentenced to seven days in solitary confinement for having tea and tobacco in her possession.

From August 1848 Bridget found herself frequently in the Cascades Female Factory. Charged with assault and sentenced to twelve months imprisonment with hard labour, when this sentence had finished, she was sent to the Brickfields, presumably waiting to be hired. While there, she was charged with tampering with the dormitory light and returned to the Factory for four months imprisonment with hard labour in the separate apartments. By January 1850, and back at the Brickfields, disorderly conduct returned her to the Factory for another two months hard labour again in the separate apartments. On the same day, this sentence was extended six months when she was found guilty of another charge of disorderly conduct. A pattern was clearly emerging and Bridget continued to play up in the Factory.

The offences continued. For knitting needles and wool in her possession in December 1850, three months imprisonment with hard labour. For being noisy in the ward in April 1851 she was sent to the separate cells. Later that month, 48 hours in solitary for looking over the door of her cell. In May of the same year, she was ordered to sleep and eat in the separate apartments for quarrelling in the mess room. Also that month, fourteen days in the separate cells for disorderly conduct. The remainder of 1851 included three days in solitary confinement and detained in separate treatment for talking in the separate apartments, cells for seven days for disorderly conduct, and fourteen days in the cells for threatening to strike a fellow prisoner. With each return to the Factory, Bridget breached regulations. She was punished for not performing her work, destroying her clothing, altering her apron, starching her cap, having tobacco in her possession, having tobacco in her mouth, idling at her work, talking in chapel and leaving the ranks. In October 1852 she was ordered to wear a black cap and short-sleeved jacket for ten days for talking in solitary confinement.

A Ticket of Leave was granted in July 1852 but this was revoked in mid-September after she was charged with disturbing the peace by fighting—for this, one month imprisonment with hard labour. Shortly after she was charged with being out after hours and received three months hard labour with a ruling that she was not to be hired in the District of Hobart.

Bridget was granted a Free Certificate in June 1853, but she continued to commit offences and appears to have moved around the colony, living under various names. In April 1859,

in the Supreme Court in Hobart, she was charged with stealing money, but was found not guilty and acquitted. In November 1860, when living at Green Ponds (now Kempton), she was sentenced to one month in prison with hard labour for being idle and disorderly, then in December 1864, living at Campbell Town, she was charged with being a common prostitute and sent to prison for one month hard labour. In July 1871, as Bridget Clark alias Brewer, she was fined ten shillings (or in default 48 hours in solitary confinement) for being drunk and incapable, and in February 1873, as Bridget Brewer, she appeared in the Police Office with George Clark. Both were fined 10 shillings for being drunk and incapable (or in default, 48 hours in prison).

Four years passed without offence, however the offending resumed when in Westbury in March 1877, as Bridget Brewer, she was sentenced to fourteen days in prison for being idle and disorderly. Twelve months later a bundle of clothing belonging to Bridget's husband was stolen from Launceston's White Hart Inn. At the time Bridget was living in Longford. The court report noted that she appeared 'stupid from the effects of drink'.

In Launceston, in February 1879, as Brewer or Murphy, Bridget was charged with vagrancy and sent to prison for fourteen days. Five months passed and she was fined 10 shillings for being drunk—the same offence and sentence repeated again in November 1885. After offending for 40 years, her last known offence was in May 1886 when, in the Launceston Police Court, she was charged with damaging a dwelling house and breaking four panes of glass valued at six shillings. Found guilty, she was ordered to pay for the damage—or to go to prison for a month.

In February 1892, as Bridget Brewer, a labourer's wife, Bridget died in hospital in Launceston from a cerebral haemorrhage and Bright's disease (a disease of the kidneys). She was 65.

SARAH
BAKER

Sarah Baker was not a woman to mess with. When she said something, she meant it. She and John Kelly lived together for six years at Totnes in Devon. John Kelly was drunk. He should have known better than to strike Sarah. She had warned him. 'Do that again and I will knock your brains out.' He did, so she did.

On 12 March 1842 Sarah faced the judge at the Devon Assizes where she was tried for wilful murder. The court heard that the pair were drunk and quarrelling in a public house. Sarah struck her partner violently on the shoulder with a poker. She then hit him with a fire shovel and her heavy nailed shoe. Sarah's defence was that she had warned him not to hit her. John lived for ten days after the assault. Sarah was found guilty of manslaughter and was transported for Life.

Sarah was baptised in 1823 in Penzance in Cornwall where her father was a shipwright. She left her three sisters and a brother behind when she sailed on the *Royal Admiral* in May 1842. The ship stopped at the Cape of Good Hope to take on fresh drinking water, and sailed into the Derwent River in late September. The female factories were full when the ship arrived so there was a seven day delay in landing the women. Many of the women were sent on to Launceston.

Before disembarkation, the women's descriptions were recorded. The scribe noted Sarah's sleepy heavy look, her long thick nose and perhaps, when he looked up, her height surprised him. She was tall at 5 feet 6 inches. Over the next couple of years, Sarah was charged with several offences for drunkenness, being absent without leave and theft. In 1847 she married John Waring, a convict who arrived on the *Coromandel* (2). Four men applied to marry Sarah. Did they know her history? Her temper? Knowingly or not, Waring married a feisty woman with a bad temper and a penchant for alcohol.

Initially, John may have considered himself lucky to marry Sarah. But he learnt quickly. In January 1848 she was sentenced to three months hard labour for abusing her husband. He was dangerously ill at the time. Sarah was returned to the Brickfields depot in March 1848 because her husband was in hospital and she had no means of support. Her daughter, Sarah Warren Baker, was born in May 1848 at the Cascades Female Factory. Shortly afterwards, John died in the New Norfolk hospital and Sarah petitioned Governor Denison for an indulgence. With her Ticket of Leave she could earn a living and support her child. However she was not granted her ticket, even though the magistrate, A.B. Jones, reminded the Governor of her great distress and of his promise to her husband to assist her. Instead, her generally bad behaviour, including the abuse of her husband and her drunken dispos-ition, worked against her. Soon after, baby Sarah died from convulsions at the Dynnyrne nursery.

Over the next four years, Sarah spent time in the Cascades, Launce-ston and Ross factories charged with drunkenness and absconding. At Ross, in 1852, she gave birth to Susannah, whose father was recorded as William Warren. Sarah's misdemeanours continued and she spent a lot of time during her daughter's infant years in and out of the factories.

Susannah was admitted to the Orphan School in 1859. She was six years old and her father was dead. She was discharged to her mother on a single occasion, but the reunion was short lived. Susannah was sent back to the orphanage and her mother to the Factory. In 1861, Sarah stole a pair of boots from a hawker in Macquarie Street. He was an old man, but determined not to lose his goods. He grabbed Sarah and she assaulted him, hitting him over the head with the boots. She did not desist even when the constabulary arrived. Once again her previous offences and history of alcohol abuse worked against her. The magistrate determined that it would be best for Sarah's child to be removed from someone with such drunken habits.

Sarah moved around the north of the state leaving her daughter's care to the authorities. In October 1865 she married Robert Salmon, a 45-year-old bachelor. Married life did not put an end to her carousing, nor did it seem to offer any stability. In July 1866 Sarah faced the magistrate again, charged with being idle and disorderly and having no visible means of support. She was supposedly in labour, but her advanced stage of pregnancy gained her no sympathy and she was sent to the gaol for fourteen days. Two days after her scheduled release, Sarah gave birth to a daughter, Mary Ann, at Deloraine.

Perhaps her father took care of Mary Ann, as Sarah was charged as idle and disorderly at Deloraine and Launceston while her child was still an infant. Again, she went back to the Factory, now the Launceston Gaol. In November 1868 advertisements appeared in the local papers searching for a Robert Salmon, late of the 11th Regiment of Infantry, who left his contingent in Van Diemen's Land in 1844. A Melbourne legal firm offered a reward for information. If this was Sarah's husband, it was almost too late for her to benefit.

Sarah died of consumption in the Westbury district on 22 May 1869. Her husband, Robert, a labourer of Exton, registered her death.

ISABELLA
MUNRO

The 'very bad' Isabella Munro, a 24-year-old needlewoman from Argyleshire, Scotland with black hair and light hazel eyes, arrived in Hobart on 10 August 1850 on board the *Aurora* (2). Transported for ten years for 'theft by opening lock fast places', this was the fourth time Isabella had been sentenced for larceny, previously having spent over five and a half years in prison.

Isabella was unmarried and literate. Her physical characteristics were fairly average, but one feature stands out—she wore a wooden leg. This characteristic certainly did not hinder Isabella's ability to wreak havoc, in fact in some instances, it was her enabler!

Between her arrival and February 1852, Isabella worked for a number of people in and around Hobart. However, on 18 February she was greeted at the Cascades Female Factory for the beginning of a six month sentence of hard labour for being absent and insolent to Mr W. Chambers, for whom she was working at Old Wharf, Hobart. Four months into her sentence, on 14 June 1852, Isabella spent three days on a diet of bread and water for disorderly conduct. Nevertheless her behaviour obviously wasn't considered poor enough to keep her inside, as just two weeks later she was working for Mr Bentley of Kelly Street, Hobart.

Four months passed and Isabella absconded for reasons unknown, and was immediately returned to the Factory on 22 October 1852 and a sentence of twelve months hard labour. Early the following year she was caught with knitting and other articles in her bed. No punishments were listed, yet disorderly conduct in the following weeks, saw another three months of hard labour tacked onto Isabella's sentence. Her penchant for being 'disorderly' during early 1853 might have been related to her reasons for absconding—we will never know for sure, but on 11 June 1853 Isabella gave birth to an illegitimate child, Mary.

After a fourteen-day stint in the separate apartments, with only one hour of exercise per day and keeping Isabella from her child, she tidied up her act. In August 1854 she was recorded as being at the Queen's Orphan School (perhaps visiting Mary) and the very next day at the Factory. Soon after she was assigned to work for S. Corrigan in Jerusalem (now Colebrook). Receiving her Ticket of Leave on 7 November 1854, Isabella applied to marry labourer Thomas Ward the following summer. They married in St James' Church, Jerusalem on 29 January 1855. Receiving her Conditional Pardon in September 1857, she and Thomas appear to have moved to Muddy Plains.

In 1860 William Finlay was charged with 'burglariously entering the dwelling of Isabella Ward ... and stealing therefrom £6., clothing belonging to her husband to the value of £5., and other articles'. This was not the end of Isabella and William meeting in the courts—in August 1862 William Finlay and John Bryan deposited an array of stolen goods from a nearby farm on Isabella's property. A court case ensued and many interesting details were revealed—first, Bryan referred to Isabella as 'Peg-Leg Ward', second, Sergeant Rose in giving evidence suggested that he 'knew that Finlay lived with Ward, but believed he was not her husband'.

After varying and contradictory statements from all, C.A.W. Rocher Esq., prosecutor on behalf of the Crown, suggested 'it was merely the falling out of thieves'. Both Bryan and Finlay were found guilty and sentenced to four years penal servitude. Meanwhile Isabella had been released from questioning only to find herself embroiled in two other cases. Charged with stealing a shawl in February 1862, the property of Jane Warlock, the case took nearly six months to reach the courts. Isabella was found guilty and sentenced to six months hard labour meaning that the other case in which Isabella was embroiled was in limbo with her unable to appear in Court. In this instance, Isabella was prosecuting Charles Jones, who was charged with stealing two blankets from her. The case was adjourned for a later date.

In mid-1863 Isabella accused Anna Quick of 'feloniously and burglariously' entering her house and stealing two of her dresses worth £2 and Anna was found guilty. The *Launceston Examiner* dated 11 June 1863 reported Anna being sentenced to nine months, a decision not made lightly. It appears the courts were becoming all too familiar with Isabella. The recorder of the case, in sentencing Anna said:

> ... that from his own knowledge of Ward's bad habits he could easily have supposed that she might, when in a state of intoxication, have given the dresses to the prisoner to take care of, and then on becoming sober, have forgotten the circumstances and charged her with stealing them.

Unfortunately for Anna, Isabella had been proven sober that night, and unlikely to have forced open her own door.

The following year was relatively quiet for Isabella, perhaps due to the death of her husband Thomas in October 1864. The couple appear to have been estranged, with Thomas serving out his long and painful illness at his son's residence in Hobart, across the State from Isabella.

In trouble again—the following October in 1865, the *Cornwall Chronicle* reported:

A BRUTAL assault was perpetrated on Friday night, on a woman of the town, named Jane Simpson, by Jane Williams, alias Tame, and Isabella Munroe, the latter a well known character with a wooden leg. The woman Simpson was near her confinement, and she received such injuries as has since endangered her life. The assault was committed near Chester's public house, in Wellington-street, where Ward kicked Simpson in the abdomen with the wooden leg, and Williams nearly bit one of her fingers off.

On 30 October Isabella and Jane appeared before the court. None of the details are reported but Isabella got off scot-free, Jane receiving a fine of 40 shillings or one month of hard labour.

In July 1866 Isabella married George Johnson in the York Street Mission House in Launceston, although not happily ever after. On 28 February 1867 George was charged with having assaulted Isabella. She declined to present to court and George was discharged. Three days later, after an argument, George attacked again, this time with a knife. The *Cornwall Chronicle* reported that Isabella 'put up her hands to save her throat, when the fellow inflicted a wound which nearly severed the four fingers from the woman's right hand'. Arriving at the scene, police took statements from Isabella, many of which she retracted in front of Police Magistrate William Gunn on 16 March. She admitted to having been drinking when the incident occurred. The truth of what happened that evening was only ever to be known by Isabella and George, however the report in the *Chronicle* concluded— 'The Bench after warning the prisoner and the woman Isabella Ward that their quarrels would terminate badly for both if they did not alter their conduct, dismissed the case and discharged the prisoner'.

What happened to Isabella and George after 1870 is unknown, although there are two deaths registered in Tasmania between 1895 and 1905 either of which may be our Isabella.

LYDIA
GORDON

Self-professed cook for the Duchess of Gloucester, Lydia Gordon was transported as a result of stealing from her employer, the exact details of which vary depending on the source. Lydia when stating her offence said 'robbing my mistress of plate value of £25', the clerk recording her prosecutor as Ruddox. The proceedings of the Central Criminal Court, 21 October 1850, states that

Lydia Gordon pleaded guilty of stealing one watch and other articles, value £37 13 shillings, the goods of Samuel Riddick in his dwelling-house. Either way Lydia received seven years and arrived in Van Diemen's Land on the *Aurora* (2) on 10 August 1851.

The surgeon's report of Lydia's behaviour on board the ship was only one word 'exemplary' and the 25-year-old, hazel-eyed brunette, upon her arrival into the colony was immediately assigned to Mr Roope of New Town. Six months into her position with Mr Roope, Lydia was recorded as visiting the hospital, but discharged the same day back to her employer. Less than two weeks later Lydia absconded, however it seems she may have had a solid reason for doing so as she is recorded as being admitted to the hospital on the same day.

In March 1852 Lydia went to work for William Thomas Napier Champ (ex-Commandant of Port Arthur) in Swanport on the east coast of Van Diemen's Land and remained in his employ until later that year when it appears she returned into the service of Mr Roope. It was from here that she was charged with 'refusing to work' in November 1852 and was sentenced to seven days in the cells at the Female Factory.

On 24 January 1853 Lydia was married to Jero Neron, a 25-year-old bachelor, at St John's in New Town—but very soon after 'her husband having gone to the diggings', it was declared on 4 February that she be returned to the government (the Factory) as she was considered as not being under suitable control. It appears that as a married woman with her husband away, Lydia struggled to focus on her work. During the next four years she was drunk, disorderly, disobedient and absent from work enough to receive over seventeen months in and out of hard labour at the Female Factory. During this time Lydia managed to be granted her Ticket of Leave three times, only to have it revoked each time!

On 17 January 1857 the *Launceston Examiner* reported on the most recent revocation:

A FEMALE ABSCONDER — Lydia Gordon, a ticket of leave servant at the Hospital, was sentenced yesterday to nine months imprisonment with hard labour for absconding from her service. A cash box was missed simultaneously with the prisoner, who had evidently taken it, though the proof was not sufficient to sustain the more serious charge.

The newspaper never followed up on Lydia's sentence but it would appear that the evidence required to support the charge of larceny was put forward, as two days later the addi-

tional charge of 'larceny under £5' was added to Lydia's record along with '18 months hard labor cumulative upon and to commence at expiration of existing sentence of hard labor'.

Amid all of the toing and froing, in June 1855, Lydia's connection with important Port Arthur officials continued when she was sent to work at Port Arthur for Mr Boyd. There were two Boyds working at Port Arthur at the time, Adolarius Humphrey Boyd (the settlement's accountant) and James Boyd, the Civil Commandant. Which of the two Lydia was working for is unknown, however this posting appeared to last about a year until she took work in Launceston for Mr Miller.

By 21 October 1857 Lydia had served out her required sentence and was Free by Servitude, receiving her Certificate of Freedom on 7 May 1858.

MARY
LEARY

Mary Leary, aged 26, was tried for murder on 30 July 1840 in County Meath and was sentenced to trans-portation for Life. A widow with two children, Mary was tried in her home county. Described as a house servant, and 5 feet 4¼ inches tall with a fair complexion, she had brown hair, blue eyes, and a freckled mole on the right side of her chin.

It seems likely that Mary brought her two children with her on the *Mary Anne* in 1841. Shortly after the ship arrived, two young boys, Thomas and James Leary, were admitted to the Queen's Orphan Schools at New Town. James remained there for twelve months and Thomas until January 1846. On the admission register, their mother's name was recorded as 'Judith Leary' but there was no woman of this name on the *Mary Anne*. Mary's surname also appears to interchange between Leary and Leavy on the colonial records however the Irish transportation register recorded her surname as Leary.

Mary was in the colony less than a year when her first application for permission to marry was submitted. Mary and Richard Neal successfully applied to marry in January 1842. The couple married the following month in St Mark's Church of England at Pontville. Mary, aged 26, was a widow, and Richard, aged 44, was a farmer and widower.

Granted a Ticket of Leave in November 1845 she managed to stay out of trouble until 1851, when, as Mary Neal, she appeared in the Richmond Quarter Sessions, charged with assault and beating Susan Loane. The *Colonial Times* reported that Susan Loane's appearance evoked 'much sympathy bearing evident tokens of a serious ill-treatment'. She was about sixteen and had lived as a servant to Mary for some eighteen months. Mary had beaten her several times with a stick, breaking her arm, and forcing her to continue to work rather than seeking treatment. As a result her arm had not set properly. At the time, Mary was living with former convict Rhody Kennedy at Brighton. Mary and Rhody were both sentenced to imprisonment, were to pay a fine of £20, were to find two sureties in £20 each to pay the fines, and to be further imprisoned until the fines were paid and sureties given. Mary was to serve her two year sentence at the House of Correction (the Cascades Female Factory). Her Ticket of Leave was also revoked, but granted again in January 1853.

It is not clear what became of Mary's husband, Richard Neal, but in May 1853, Mary and Rhody Kennedy, then free, applied for permission to marry. Approval was apparently given but Mary was back before the courts before a marriage could take place. In June 1853 she was sentenced to nine months imprisonment with hard labour with an additional nine months probation for being absent all night from her place of residence. Her Ticket of Leave was revoked again in August 1853, but reinstated in October 1854.

Granted permission to reside in the District of Richmond in January 1855, in March the following year Mary and Phillip Whelan, a former convict but by then free, successfully applied for permission to marry. They married later that month, on 24 March, in a Church of England service in the 'Government Chapel Township of Colebrook Dale', in the District of Richmond. Mary was a widow aged 37 and Phillip a labourer aged 34. At the end of November 1856 her Conditional Pardon was approved.

Mary may have died in 1872 in hospital in Hobart, aged 51. Philip Whelan, an Irish-born labourer aged 60, died of pneumonia in hospital in Hobart in September 1874. He was buried in a pauper grave at Corne-lian Bay cemetery. They had at least one son—John Philip Whelan, born in 1857 in Richmond District.

REBECCA
DAYNES

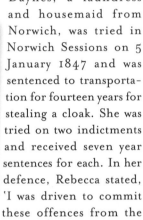

Rebecca Daynes, a laundress and housemaid from Norwich, was tried in Norwich Sessions on 5 January 1847 and was sentenced to transporta-tion for fourteen years for stealing a cloak. She was tried on two indictments and received seven year sentences for each. In her defence, Rebecca stated, 'I was driven to commit these offences from the ill-treatment of my husband'. Rebecca, however, had been convicted of similar offences twice before and she was described as 'a thief for many years'. She had two previous periods of imprisonment in Norwich.

Rebecca Daynes (née Simmons) arrived in Van Diemen's Land on the *Asia* (7) on 21 July 1847 with her baby son, Edward. The *Asia* (7) brought 170 women. They spent their first six months on the hulk *Anson* moored in the River Derwent, separated from what was believed to be the contam-inating influence of the 'old hands', and receiving training to fit them for their new life as domestic servants in the colony.

At the time of her transportation Rebecca was 28 and married with three children. As with many convict women, she wore simple tattoos—a ring and five blue dots on her finger. In many cases, the meaning of the tattoos has been lost. Some were created during the voyage, etched into the skin with soot and black sediment from lamps.

Rebecca's indent noted that her husband James, father Joseph, mother Mary Ann and siblings George, Charles, Emily and Ruth were all living at Norwich. Two of her children remained behind in Norwich and went to live with their maternal grandparents, Joseph and Mary Simmons or Samons.

In May 1850 Rebecca gave birth to a child, Annie, at the Cascades Female Factory. Annie lived only nine days, dying in the Factory on 23 May from *erysipelas,* a serious and contagious skin disease. Rebecca's infant son who came with her on the *Asia* was admitted to the Queen's Orphan School as Edward Deans, on 1 July 1851 when he was four years four months old. He transferred from the infant section of the Orphan School to the Male Orphan School in December 1854. He remained there until July 1862, when he was apprenticed in Hobart.

Rebecca made two applications for permission to marry, both to fellow convicts. The first, in July 1849, was to convict Peter Miller, who arrived

on the *Abercrombie* in 1841. It was refused—no reason for the refusal was recorded. The second was approved, in September 1851, to convict James Howes, who arrived on the *Equestrian* (1) in 1844. The couple married on 13 October 1851 in St George's Church of England, Sorell. James 'Hewes', aged 28, was an illiterate labourer. Rebecca was described as a widow aged 29. She signed her name with her mark 'X'.

In January 1852, not long after she had married, pregnant Rebecca absconded and was found on board the *Pilot* bound for Victoria. Her attempted escape was to have a tragic outcome— she was sentenced to eighteen months imprisonment with hard labour in the Cascades Female Factory. While there, in March 1852, she gave birth to a stillborn child. Was the father of the child Peter Miller with whom she had applied for permission to marry 8 months earlier? And why was she seeking to escape from the colony, leaving her husband? About a fortnight later, Rebecca died at the Factory.

An inquest into Rebecca's death was held on 31 March 1852, in the 'dead house' at the Factory. A.B. Jones, Coroner, determined that she died from consumption or *phthisis pulmonalis.*

In 1893, 43 years after Rebecca's death, the *Brisbane Courier* published the following in its 'Missing Friends' column:

DAYNES, Rebecca, left Norwich in 1846 for Hobart, Tasmania, taking her baby with her. Her son Walter longs for news of her (father is dead).

MARY

SHAW

'Never used to any work—quite useless as a servant' and 'an old thief' was how Mary Shaw was described in her gaol report and record. Mary was convicted at the Stafford Quarter Sessions on 15 October 1828, and sentenced to seven years transportation for stealing a watch from a person. Her record suggests that she had been convicted previously of a similar crime and was not necessarily a solo act being 'connected with a gang of thieves'.

Aged 32 when the *Lady of the Lake* departed Woolwich in June 1829, Mary stood at 4 feet 9¼ inches, had a dark complexion and grey eyes and a deep scar in the centre of her forehead. She was a native of Church Easton in Staffordshire and a widow, her husband Thomas Shaw had passed away before she was transported. Mary could read but not write and claimed to be a farm servant. All of these attributes and details were made clear in both Mary's trial and subsequent documentation. However, when Mary stepped on board that vessel, bound for Van Diemen's Land, she had one secret that no-one knew ... she was balding!

Just five days after setting sail on 19 June 1829, Mary was admitted on the sick list with *tinea capitis*. In the surgeon's notes he wrote that Mary had 'endeavoured to conceal [her condition] for some motive or other'. *Tinea capitis* is an infection caused by a fungi of scalp hair follicles and the surrounding skin. The condition is usually contracted by people from personal contact with other people suffering from the infection or from dogs or cats.

From where Mary contracted this terrible condition is unknown, but it was well advanced by the time she boarded the ship and was only discovered after an examination by the surgeon following complaints by her 'mess-mates' who suggested that she was 'being very offensive'. On examination the surgeon found Mary was in fact wearing 'false hair and her head in a most filthy state; the disease having reached its very acme from sheer neglect'.

The surgeon went on to suggest that what little hair Mary had left, she had cut close and that shaving was out of the question due to the 'aggravated state' of her condition. She received several treatments on board including *Unguentum Sulphuris*—or sulphur ointment. Mary remained on the sick list for nearly two months, being finally discharged on 9 August.

The *Lady of the Lake* docked in Hobart on 1 November 1829, and presumably shortly afterwards Mary was assigned as a servant. Her first recorded discretion, was 'neglect of duty' reported by her master Mr Trenery for which Mary was returned to the 'Service of the Crown' and not to be assigned for two months. During this time, Mary would have worked within the walls of the Female Factory, however in May 1833—while working for a master named Makepeace—Mary was charged with being absent without leave and returned to the Female Factory to spend one month at the wash tub. Some two months later Mary was absent without leave again, although this time she was found 'in bed with a man' in what the authorities considered a disorderly house! This time it was two months at the wash tub, hard labour at the best of times not to mention in the depths of winter. She was also sentenced to sleep 'in a cell' at night.

Having completed her two months on the tub, Mary obviously felt the need to celebrate when assigned to her new master, because after 'having been liberated from the Factory only 14 days she is to be placed in the C. [Crime] Class' she was charged with

being drunk and disorderly. For this, Mary was not to be assigned in Hobart Town—an attempt to free her of the temptations of the town?

Away from temptations, Mary served out the rest of her sentence and became Free by Servitude in October 1835 receiving her Certificate of Freedom. The final note recorded on Mary's conduct record is another conviction in 1842, although the actual crime is not recorded. Her sentence is listed as seven years and after serving some fourteen months Mary received her Ticket of Leave.

Mary applied to marry free man Thomas Gibson in November 1845, and in January 1846 she and Thomas were wed. Whether their life together was happy, we will never know, but after 22 years together, Mary passed away age 60 at Oyster Cove on 9 April 1868 from diarrhoea.

CATHERINE OWENS

Catherine Owens arrived in Van Diemen's Land as a young woman with attitude. When she was sentenced in March 1829 to fourteen years transportation for receiving stolen goods, 'the hardened offender' (aged 19) 'dropped a curtsy, and impudently said, "Thank you, my Lord".'

Almost a decade later she stood

before a country court on the other side of the world. She was an assigned servant, working without pay, and yet she infuriated her master by stating her own terms and conditions of employment.

She had arrived tipsy at her most recent assignment to Mr Richard Willis, owner of a large property in the Midlands. 'After dinner', Willis told the court, 'the prisoner sent for me, and said unless she was allowed to smoke she would not stop, that she could not do without it. I said I would allow no such thing. Then, she replied, "I won't stop".'

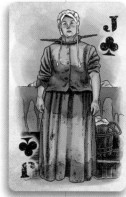

Ten years in the convict system of Van Diemen's Land including a sentence of three days in an iron collar had done nothing to reform 'Cath' Owens. Instead, she had made a place for herself as a member of a network of convict women who would rather spend their time together in a Female Factory than serve the settlers. These women had become notorious in the Cascades Female Factory as the Flash Mob.

They ruled the Crime Class Yard. Their allegiances were to each other, and they treated the rules and regulations of the convict system with disdain. Cath and her friends created for themselves a vibrant world within the prison walls. Their drab uniforms were transformed into stylish dress.

Their caps were embroidered, they wore rings in their ears, and swirled their silk scarves. With plenty of time on their hands, they told stories, sang songs, and made up their own plays, complete with costumes.

But there was also a dark side to the Flash Mob. They intimidated other women, as a fellow prisoner in the Launceston Female Factory, Eliza Churchill, told a governmental committee of enquiry in May 1842. By this time Cath and her friends had been sent north to break the nexus of relationships, but they simply regrouped and continued as before, except that their sexuality now became an issue.

'There are many women', testified Eliza Churchill, 'who will not stay out of the Factory when others with whom they carry on an unnatural connexion are in the building'. Eliza named six couples, including Catherine Owens and Ellen Scott. 'The other women are afraid to interfere although they dislike such practices, they are never carried on openly but at night, they are never associated with by the other women, they generally sit together on one side of the yard.' During the day there is little for them to do, they 'amuse themselves the best way they can, dancing & singing etc'.

Confident and cocky, they believed

they could manipulate the system, and Eliza had heard them say that 'if any attempt were made to separate the women whose names I have mentioned & others of similar habits a riot would be got up immediately, I heard Ellen Scott say so last night if Catherine Owens were sent to Hobarton'. These women had thoroughly frightened the superintendent in charge of the Factory. 'At present', he said in his own statement to the governmental enquiry, 'if anything is wrong it is dangerous to go among the large number in one room. If I need to take a prisoner out of the Crime Class, the others defy me, & I am obliged to carry pistols, I have had my shirt torn from my back. In almost every case I am obliged to use force to take a woman out as they will seldom come out when called, but call the others to their assistance'.

Eliza Churchill and the superintendent offered their warning testimony in May 1842 and in October that year a riot was indeed 'got up' on behalf of Cath Owens. As a Convict Department official would later report to his superiors in Hobart Town, the problem began when Cath, 'an extremely bad character, and one who has always ranked as a leader upon all occasions of misconduct', was locked into a solitary cell to serve a sentence for absconding. In the afternoon when a matron came to check on the prisoner, she was seized by Cath's friends. Cath was liberated, and

the 85 women in the Crime Class Yard 'bid defiance to the authorities in the Factory, one and all stating they would not allow her to serve the remainder of her sentence in the Cells'.

The siege continued all night and into the next day, until 30 police, joined by 30 male convicts and armed with sledgehammers and crowbars, 'made a breach through the wall, and came to close quarters with their Amazonian captives. The women fought like demons' but 'were finally overcome by superior strength, and compelled to capitulate'.

Back Cath went to Hobart Town, back to the Cascades Female Factory where the Flash Mob started. There a new yard of 'separate apartments' awaited women just like her. Under the regime made possible by these double-storey blocks of cells, prisoners could be kept in silence, totally isolated from each other. No Flash Mob could exist under these conditions, and Catherine Owens, who was still in the system after thirteen years, could no longer spend days with friends dancing and singing in style.

ELIZABETH PAYNE

Nothing marks Elizabeth Payne out as special except an undelivered letter to her husband. From public records,

Elizabeth looks like just another poor woman who pawned what she stole for a bit of money. On 17 October 1826 she was tried and convicted at the Devon Quarter Sessions in her native Exeter. Sentenced to seven years transportation, Elizabeth was shipped off to Van Diemen's Land on the *Persian* (1), reaching her destination on 5 August 1827. Told by a colonial official to state her crime in her own words, she said 'Stealing in my lodgings and pledging (pawning) a blanket'. And then she added for the record that she was married, 'Husband on board the Java, a Private Marine', or as she may have explained more fully, my husband is a private in the Royal Marines, the infantry land-fighting division of the Royal Navy.

From Elizabeth's convict conduct record we know that for the most part she spent her years under sentence doing exactly what she was told. Only twice in seven years did she indulge in impulsive behaviour. The first time was in the winter of 1829 when she was working at the Male Orphan School and was ordered one Sunday to chaperone the boys as they walked to St David's—this was before the purpose-built orphanage at New Town made going to church a simple matter of moving from one building to another on the same site. On their way home Elizabeth was lured away from the path of righteousness, and later charged with 'absenting herself from the children on their road from Church yesterday and remaining absent until near 4 o'clock and being intoxicated'. Her punishment was a trip to the newly opened Cascades Female Factory for a week of confinement in a solitary cell, an experience she took care not to repeat.

For almost three years she is invisible because her record is spotless. Then in January 1832 Elizabeth was charged with being 'drunk and insolent to her Mistress', though the insolence must have been fairly mild because she was reprimanded without further punishment. On 17 October 1833, exactly seven months after her trial, Elizabeth received a certificate to say that she was free.

None of this tells us very much about her except that she understood where power lay and tried as a prisoner to move inconspicuously through the convict system. But who was she as an individual with a life outside the system? For most model prisoners such as Elizabeth—and there were many—that question is unanswerable. Only by a fluke does the undelivered letter to her husband survive to bring her for a moment into sharper focus.

Composing a letter was clearly an ordeal for Elizabeth, who wrote English as she heard it, and not according to the standard rules of spelling and punctuation followed by confidently literate people. 'Dear husbent i ham happy to inform you that we arrivd hear yesterday'. Most of the passengers were probably eager to leave the ship after almost four months at sea, but not Elizabeth. As long as she was on the *Persian* she had not been totally cut adrift from the global network of the Royal Navy to which she belonged as the wife of a marine, 'i hope the Lord will stand my freand for i have none hear with me only the Doctor and the officers on board the behave very well to us on our passage'. It was to the officers that she was entrusting this letter, this gesture to keep her connected to her husband.

As for the man himself, her feelings were deeply conflicted. After a conventional greeting wishing him well and in good health, she switches abruptly to accusation, 'whet ever i goe throu i shell say you was the Cause ofit and thet you very well kno i ham bound to Curse the Day that i ever saw stonehouse or any init'. It is, 'with a aching hart', writes Elizabeth, 'thet I thank on the wishes you Leid on me when you was in the hospital'. And what were these 'wishes'? Pipe dreams of an alluring life? Had William Payne wooed his wife in a military hospital when he was recovering from wounds or illness?

Whatever he had promised, he had badly let her down, and seems to have got himself into some sort of trouble which tarnished his reputation, 'i hope you will not return to Plymouth thet no one will Cast any reflections on you'. Plymouth, about 70 kilometres southwest of Elizabeth's hometown of Exeter, was the coastal port where companies from the Royal Marines were often stationed. Whatever happened there may have been the cause, as far as Elizabeth was concerned, of her theft from her lodgings and her subsequent sentence to exile, 'but i forgive you' she writes, 'and i hope the Lord will is the prayers of your Distresed wife'.

This letter is more than a curse upon her husband's head. Elizabeth wants her marriage back again, wants the connectedness to someone else in the world. She tells William that she doesn't know where she will be sent 'but i hope i shell goe to Service intill my time [is] up then i will return home'. Or, here is another possibility—'if you Can Come to me I wish you would'. Fearful, perhaps, of stepping onto the unknown shores of Van Diemen's Land, this 29-year-old woman tried to imagine a future in which she might re-connect with the familiar past of 'home' and marriage, though neither had been kind to her. She was on her own now, and would have to make do the best she could.

MARY
HUTCHINSON

Mary Hutchinson spent more time inside Australia's female factories than any other woman. She was just a small child when her father Francis Oakes was appointed Super-intendent of the Parra-matta Female Factory, and perhaps she thought she was escaping the world of prison administration when she married a man more than twice her age and sailed with him to Tonga. John Hutchinson, the first Wesleyan minis-ter ordained in Australia, needed a wife if he was to be a missionary, and Francis Oakes had plenty of daughters to choose from (five of the first six Oakes children were girls), including sixteen-year-old Mary.

Mary was unprepared for the dour life of Methodist missionaries, one of whom dismissed her in his private journal as 'very young and inconsiderate, she laughs very much' and 'is very worldly'. Two years in Tonga changed all that. In the surviving images of Mary Hutchinson, nothing is visible of the worldly laughing bride. Life ground Mary into a prison matron.

Ill-health released the Hutchin-sons from Tonga after John was deemed 'very weakly and unfit for so trying a place'. He was clearly a strange man, and his diffi-cult personality was dramatically on display in the confines of a missionary station. Opinion was polarised in the congregation when he was eventually sent to Hobart's Melville Street Wesleyan Chapel, after almost two years recu-perating in New South Wales. What Hutchinson's successor would call a 'Spirit of disaffection' had 'crept into the Church' and 'done much mischief' during Hutchinson's brief tenure. He seems to have been forced out, though he had his supporters, and some left the congregation, 'because they regarded my prede-cessor as an injured man'.

On 4 January 1832 John and Mary Hutchinson took up appointments as Superintendent and Matron of the Female Factory at Cascades. They had been married almost six years. Mary, now 22 years old, had given birth to four children. The first, born in Tonga, died after their return to New South Wales. The fourth would die three months after the Hutchinsons moved into rooms above the Female Factory's entryway. These rooms, overlooking the prison, would be their home for the next nineteen years. Here Mary would give birth to another eight children, and the unhealthy conditions of the Female Factory would afflict them, just as it did the children of the incarcerated convicts. The last of the four or five Hutchinson children to die in the Factory was nine-year-old Elizabeth whose death from 'disease of the brain' came only months before her parents finally departed their gloomy abode.

If Mary Hutchinson performed all the tasks set out for her as Matron, she must have left her own children in the care of convict servants for hours at a time. According to the regulations, the Matron's day began early: 'She is to inspect the Females in their separate wards at the morning muster, and shall see that they are clean and properly dressed'. She must also inspect 'the sleeping rooms daily, and see that they are kept perfectly clean and in order by the Wardswomen'. She must make sure that work was progressing apace, giving 'instructions to the Task-women about the employment of the Females' and receiving in return 'the Articles manufactured'. She must visit 'constantly throughout the day' the Hospital, Nursery, and Kitchen yards 'to superintend and give directions in all that is going forward in either, most watchfully observing that in everything extreme cleanliness, and order, and industry, and economy prevail'. And, more generally, her

duty is to assist the Superintendent 'in the care and control of the Establishment'.

Altogether a thankless job. Too much to do. And Mary Hutchinson had neither training nor experience in running a big complex institution. However there are signs in the early years of care and dedication. Each morning, according to the convict overseer of the nursery in 1834, 'the milk for the children is served out by Mrs Hutchinson herself' ensuring that every child was nourished. Nevertheless, the badly ventilated, overcrowded nursery was notorious for sickness and death. In 1838 when the local press campaigned against conditions leading to the death of a child from apparent neglect, the *Colonial Times* railed against the Matron—'where was Mrs Hutchinson—herself a mother—all this time?' Giving birth to her eighth child was one answer, though not an explanation to satisfy the critics who also blamed her for not selecting good reliable servants for their households. Over the years, she may have hardened herself to the attacks, and lowered her expectations simply to managing the circumstances presented through the ever-changing policies and practices of the convict system.

In 1851 the Lieutenant-Governor of Van Diemen's Land reported to the colonial authorities in London that 'for some time past Mr Hutchinson's health had been such as to prevent his being of any real service in the Establishment', leaving Mary 'virtually the Superintendent'. And yet, instead of recommending that she be appointed Superintendent in her husband's stead, the Lieutenant-Governor recommended that the 'still competent' Matron be transferred to run a smaller female factory at Launceston. Her appointment could save money by amalgamating the existing positions of Superintendent and Matron into a single position. In the final days of transportation Mary Hutchinson became the sole woman appointed to manage a female factory in her own right. But because she was a woman, the position was called 'Matron'.

MARGARET SHAW

Margaret Shaw was tried at the Old Bailey on 14 September 1840 and pleaded guilty to stealing a coat valued at 10 shillings. She claimed that she was charged with pledging (pawning) clothes and that she had never been convicted before.

Her native place was recorded as the East Indies, which we now would probably and broadly call South East Asia. Margaret's story is full of unanswered questions—how did her family come to be in the East Indies? Why was she in London at the time of her trial and how long had she been there?

Margaret was 46 when she embarked, a poor widow with eight children, none of whom sailed with her. Of florid complexion, she was 5 feet 5 inches tall, stout-made, with brown to grey hair, a broad forehead, large eyebrows and dark brown eyes. A formidable appearance perhaps?

Margaret was one of 180 women who sailed on the convict transport *Rajah*, a voyage famous for the quilt which was crafted on board and which is now in the National Gallery of Australia. During the voyage, Margaret was employed in the hospital and was said by the surgeon to be 'very good' in this role. Perhaps not surprisingly when she arrived in the colony in July 1841 she was sent to the Cascades Female Factory as a nurse. She was still there two years later—in July 1843, she gave evidence at the inquest into the death of her ship-mate Mary Brown.

In October 1843 Margaret was granted a Ticket of Leave. In August the following year, the Comptroller-General recommended that she be appointed Infant

Nurse at the Female Orphan School at New Town, on a salary of £18 per annum plus a personal ration. Captain Booth, in submitting Margaret's name for the vacancy, stated, 'she appears to understand the duties and bears good testimonials'. She received recommendations from John Hutchinson, who was Superintendent of the Cascades Female Factory as well as the Assistant Colonial Surgeon. Superintendent Hutchinson pointed out that Margaret had been nurse and midwife at the Cascades Female Factory for three years, and that she was 'exceedingly well conducted' and was 'a most suitable person for the care of Children, especially in time of Sickness'.

She remained as infant nurse until November 1844, when she was appointed to a position in charge of the laundry at the Orphan Schools. No doubt Margaret, with her large hands and solid build, was considered capable and reliable. What little evidence there is suggests that she remained in charge of the laundry until September 1847, when she became Free by Servitude.

Margaret's story is an unfinished one—she disappears from the records once she was free.

ELIZABETH FERGUSON

Elizabeth Ferguson, a pickpocket from Devonport, England was tried in Devon Exeter Quarter Sessions on 2 July 1844 for stealing a watch from the person and sentenced to transportation for ten years. It was her first conviction but she had been three weeks 'on the town'.

A nursemaid aged sixteen, Elizabeth arrived on the *Tasmania* (1) five days before Christmas Day 1844. The surgeon on board the ship described her as 'dirty'. Elizabeth was only 4 feet 10 inches tall, with a brown complexion, brown hair and blue eyes. Her face was slightly pock-pitted.

Her first colonial offence was in December 1847 when she was sentenced to ten days solitary confinement for being absent from the service of her master, Giblin. Six months later, in July 1848, Elizabeth, then aged 23, married John Farrell, a clerk aged 41. They were married in St George's Church of England, Battery Point by Rev. H.P. Fry. It seems that marriage was not a settling influence on Elizabeth, although she behaved well enough to be granted a Ticket of

Leave in January 1850. After this, her behaviour deteriorated significantly.

In June 1850 Elizabeth was found in a common brothel lying on a bed with a man. For this, she was sentenced to three months imprisonment with hard labour in the Cascades Female Factory and her Ticket of Leave was revoked. In October 1850, while assigned to her husband, she was again found in a common brothel, earning her a six month stint with hard labour in the Factory. In August 1851, still assigned to her husband, she was found out after hours and was sent to the Factory for one month with hard labour.

By February 1852 she had regained her Ticket of Leave but abused the privilege when she was found in a public house in company with a sailor and with a common prostitute. She was sent to the Factory for six months with hard labour and was punished for neglect of duty while there. In January 1853, and again in October of the same year, she was sentenced to nine months imprisonment with hard labour for not only being out after hours but also being a common prostitute. In February 1853, while in the Factory, she was admonished for loud talk and laughter while at exercise.

Elizabeth received her Free Certificate in July 1854, almost ten years to the day after she was originally sentenced to transportation.

It is not known what happened to her after she served her sentence, although she may have left the colony. In Melbourne, in September 1862, a woman named Eliza Ferguson and a man were charged with making a disturbance in a house of ill-fame and annoying the neighbourhood. Both were fined five shillings. Shortly after, Eliza Ferguson was also charged with robbery. Seven years later, in August 1869, a woman named Elizabeth Ferguson, described as a disorderly prostitute, was brought before the City Police Court in Melbourne charged with making a disturbance in the street. This woman was frequently before the Courts and associated with prostitution and brothels.

MELORINA FLORENTINA DE SAUMAREZ

In 1846 nineteen-year-old Melorina Florentina de Saumarez was arrested in England, in such exciting circumstances that the event was widely reported. One journalist was particularly thrilled by her fashionable clothes and her magnificent black hair. Wholly unconfined (ladies *never* wore their hair unconfined in public), it flowed over her shoulders down to her waist.

Melorina stated that her father had been a colonel of artillery, commanding a regiment, but had died 20 years earlier. She had been born in Paris, where her mother and brother still lived, and she had received a superior education. It sounded aristocratic, and the de Saumarez were certainly a notable family in Guernsey, but as Melorina later stated that her real name was La Lausse, her relationship with them sounds doubtful.

Melorina's story was that she had arrived in Southampton from Guernsey two months earlier, on the way to visit her mother in Paris. Her claim to be the niece of Lady de Saumarez, and her ladylike deportment and fascinating manners, meant that a respectable landlady readily rented her an apartment. Melorina became friendly with a local girl, Elizabeth Purkis, daughter of a well-to-do merchant. Elizabeth invited Melorina to stay with her family.

One day Melorina said she had a severe headache, and went upstairs to lie down. The family assumed she would remain in her bedroom, but it had a door that led to Mr Purkis's bedroom. Rashly, he kept his cash box under his pillow. Several hours later Melorina left the house, carrying a small basket that appeared heavy.

She bought a matching cash box, returned, exchanged the boxes, and left the house for good.

After the robbery was discovered, Melorina was found and arrested. She did not deny the crime, but said vehemently, 'Don't let the world know I am a de Saumarez'. She sounds like an inept criminal, for she gave the money to a third party, who returned it to Purkis—the sum of £135 in cash, £99 in a cheque, and some coins, totalling the large amount of £250. Did Mr Purkis put it in a bank this time?

Three months after the arrest, Melorina was tried at the Winchester County sessions at Manchester. This time dressed demurely in black, with a black veil. The romantic circumstances of the crime aroused deep interest. It was reported, 'The fact of the prisoner being a Frenchwoman had created considerable sympathy on her behalf,' and several benevolent ladies offered help. Melorina was found guilty, and the jury recommended mercy, but the chairman said there were no extenuating circumstances. He had seldom seen a case where the advantages of education had been applied to such deep-laid schemes of vice. He sentenced Melorina to transportation for ten years. She fainted.

Melorina was sent to prison to await her transportation. She left England in March 1847 on the *Asia* (7), arriving in Hobart in July. There she was described as single, aged 20 and Catholic. She could read and write in French, and she was a needle-woman—perhaps not the way she had earned her living before, but a job she could perform in the colony as an assigned servant. She spent six months on the *Anson* serving her probation, which was extended by a week, for an unknown reason—she must have broken some minor rule.

At the beginning of 1848 Melorina would have started work as a domestic servant, but not for long. In December that year she married William King in St John's Church, Hobart. Married convict women were usually assigned to their husbands, and to all intents and purposes Melorina was free. But she could not bear Van Diemen's Land—perhaps it was the lack of soph-istication, the poverty, her husband William or domesticity—and in 1849 she tried to leave the colony. She hid on a ship, the *Duchess of Clarence*, bound for the recently discovered goldfields of California, but outgoing ships from Hobart were thoroughly searched to find runaway convicts, and Melorina was discovered. The ship's name was to be her last link with the aristocracy.

As a punishment for trying to abscond, Melorina was required to serve solitary confinement for three weeks, but after that her convict record is blank. Presumably at some stage she became free. She died in Hobart in 1876, aged 63, in poverty, and was buried in the pauper section of the cemetery. How she spent the inter-vening 26 years is unknown, but she obviously did not accumulate wealth.

HONORAH SULLIVAN

4

Honorah Sullivan was tried in her native place, County Cork, on 18 September 1851 and was sentenced to transportation for Life for commit-ting arson. She stated her offence to be 'burning a house'.

Honorah was one of 248 women transported from Ireland for arson—seven per cent of all women transported to Van Diemen's Land and a rate much higher than other groups (including Irish men) who committed this crime. Many admitted to committing arson in order to be transported but there is no evidence that Honorah did this. At the time she set fire to a house, Ireland was suffering from the dislocation, poverty and hardship caused by the aftermath of the Great Famine. This was not Honorah's first offence. According to her gaol report, she had three previous convictions, including three months for stealing clothes.

Her indent tells us that Honorah's

living relatives were her two brothers, Michael and John. John was transported for fifteen years.

Single, Roman Catholic and illiterate, she arrived on 1 September 1852 on the *Martin Luther*. There was another woman of the same name on the ship, and occasionally their records were muddled—even though they were called Honorah Sullivan 1st and Honorah Sullivan 2nd to distinguish between them. To add to the confusion, Honorah Sullivan 2nd was also from Cork and at twenty was roughly the same age as Honorah Sullivan 1st the focus of our attention here.

A housemaid aged 23, Honorah was 5 feet 3¾ inches tall with a dark complexion, dark brown hair, black eyebrows, dark eyes and a small head. She also had freckles and a scrofula mark on her left cheek and neck.

On Christmas Eve 1852 she was charged with disobedience of orders and was sentenced to four months hard labour at the Cascades Female Factory. While there, on 2 January 1853, she was accused of breaking a hair comb and despite denying having the comb she was sent to the cells for ten days. She was initially assigned in Hobart but could not keep out of trouble for long. In May she was found guilty of being absent

without leave and was sentenced to two months hard labour. In November, she refused to be assigned and was discharged to the Government. However after this she settled down and had no more colonial offences.

Honorah Sullivan and James Reilly or Riley applied for permission to marry in October 1853, but Honorah had to serve another six months before it could be approved. They applied again in February 1854, marrying on 28 February in St Joseph's Roman Catholic Church, Hobart. She was listed as a servant, aged 23 and James was a widower and farmer aged 31. He was free at the time of the marriage, having received a Conditional Pardon in December 1853. A farm labourer, James had arrived as a convict on the *London* (2) in May 1851, tried in County Mayo for stealing sheep. At the time of his transportation he was married but this does not seem to have been an impediment to his colonial marriage.

Honorah was granted a Ticket of Leave on 19 August 1856 and was recommended for a Conditional Pardon in September 1857. This was granted in June 1858. The fate of her husband James cannot be confirmed, but a farmer James Reilly passed away at Geeveston on 27 December

1892, age 75 of general debility. But Honorah, a much loved grandmother, died on 7 June 1911 at Geeveston. Her granddaughters placed a memorial notice in *The Mercury* two years later, under the name 'Hannorah Riley'.

MARY
MURPHY

The Cascades Female Factory was in its final, most austere phase when Mary Murphy entered in late September 1852 to serve a sentence of six months hard labour for 'encouraging men on her master's premises for some unlawful purpose'. The Factory now spread all the way down Degraves Street, five massive courtyards enclosed within high stone walls, an institution for a thousand women and children. The Factory was being modernised, and there was even a new bathhouse where Mary was sent to be well 'cleansed' in cold water before she put on the uniform of a prisoner.

The clean prisoner was then taken into Yard 3 where two blocks of double-tiered cells ran in parallel, with an exercise yard on each side. The blocks were segregated by religion, Protestants in one and Catholics—including Irish Mary—in the other. Mary would spend the first half of her six months punishment in a separate apartment. The Fact-

ory's Superintendent, J.M. May, was convinced that there was no better way to reform female convicts than through 'a fixed period of separate confinement, combined as in this establishment with constant application to labour; not only from the salutary dread of punishment which it inspires, but the opportunity it affords for training the minds of the prisoners to habits of obedience and industry'.

Gone was the camaraderie of the old days when women milled around in the Crime Class Yard, chatting and singing and generally making a racket. Under the regime of separate confinement, all was silent. And frightening. Mary Murphy's cell, like the other 111 cells, had two doors, 'the inner one of which is bolted, and the other one locked'. Mary slept at the end of the cell behind the bolted door, her bedding a straw mattress with a rug and two blankets. Each morning when the bell rang, she was required to fold her bedding neatly. When the outer door was unlocked and the inner door unbolted, Mary took the bedding outside. She also carried out her chamber pot, emptied and washed it, and twice a week watched as it was purified with lime.

Then back inside she went, behind the locked door. Above the door, a window space with iron grating let in enough light for her to do whatever task was set that day, mostly picking wool, sometimes hair or oakum. After she had served her three months in the separate apartment, she could look forward to a less constricted life in another Yard with more interesting tasks, perhaps needlework, or carding and spinning wool, or reeling yarn (the satisfying work of actually weaving was reserved for male prisoners). Even if she faced the really exhausting work at the laundry, there would be opportunities to chat, to be sociable. Until then, she was cooped inside this tiny cell all day, let out only for an hour of exercise walking round and round, keeping her distance from the prisoner in front and the prisoner behind, always in silence, and always under the eye of a guard. Life was very, very boring.

Sometimes Mary could not help calling attention to herself. One of the male overseers decided that her apartment was dirty (did he have it in for the Irish?), and she spent the next three days on bread and water. And then after she had been in the cells for two months she got into trouble with another overseer for talking at dinner time. What did the gaolers expect? Even behind locked and bolted doors, the women were 'positively forbidden to sing, read aloud, or make any other noise

in their apartment'. After a while your throat would seize up, your vocal chords atrophy. It wasn't possible to make no sound at all after a lifetime of talking.

Mary's only release from Yard 3 came on Sundays when she went to chapel. For a change, the prisoners actually walked together. The temptation was too great for her. On 13 December 1852, when her three months in the separate cells were nearing an end, Mary was charged with 'talking coming from chapel'. Her punishment was not to go to chapel at all the next Sunday, and instead to remain locked in her cell on bread and water.

Nothing about Mary's story suggests that she was a hardened criminal. She was in her mid-twenties when she was exiled from County Cork, where she had always lived. Her crime was stealing two sheep. Once before she had served time for stealing beef. Mary was nothing much to look at, with missing front teeth and a scar on her chin. When she sailed on the *Maria* (2) in April 1849 the ship's indent said she was married, her husband 'William in America 12 months from me'. The indent recorded two children, though they did not come with her and may have stayed in Ireland with their grandmother, also named Mary. In Van Diemen's Land her record said she was a widow and did not mention children.

After arriving in Hobart in July 1849 Mary Murphy was sent to the *Anson* for six months probation. Her first experience of the Cascades Female Factory came when she refused to work for a master, and was sentenced to a month hard labour. From there back to the Brickfields Hiring Depot where she was punished once for having a pipe in her possession, and once for smoking. The people who hired her never kept her long, and while she was under sentence, she seems to have made little or no effort in her role as convict housemaid.

In 1853, four years after Mary arrived in the penal colony, convict transportation came to an end. Moving the existing convicts quickly through the system suited local authorities keen to create a new identity for the once-dreaded island, and Mary was granted a Ticket of Leave in September 1853, less than halfway through her 10-year sentence, and in spite of her less than perfect behaviour. On 28 February 1854 an entry on her conduct record noted approval of marriage to Joseph Clegg. Though no marriage was registered, the couple may have made a life together—which would explain why the only other entries for Mary Murphy note a recommendation for a Conditional Pardon on 19 September 1854, and approval on 17 July 1855. It looks as if Mary at last had someone to talk to, and could smoke her pipe in peace.

6 GRACE HEINBURY

Grace Heinbury had a story to tell. In the autumn of 1842, four years after she arrived in Van Diemen's Land, a government committee inquiring into 'female convict prison discipline' rounded off its hearings by inviting five women to talk about their lives as prisoners. In contrast to the other witnesses, they were not actually called before the committee. A clerk took down these rare convict narratives that survive today among the unpublished papers of the committee's final report.

Grace began her story in the north of England. 'I was confined in Leicester Gaol', she said, 'and was strictly kept there, it was very well. We received instructions there from a Schoolmaster. I learned to read and write my name.' She says nothing about being arrested with a fourteen-year-old boy for stealing a piece of cheese, a pound of butter, and 'a variety of other articles'. The boy was acquitted but 26-year-old Grace was sentenced to seven years transportation.

In September 1838 Grace travelled down to London to sail on the *Atwick*. Apparently she made a good impression because 'I was appointed as Matron on board the Ship and had to look after the other Prisoners. I believe I gave satisfaction to the Surgeon Superintendent as I was well recommended when I came to Hobart Town'. That explains why she was sent to the elite household of a Supreme Court judge. 'I liked this situation,' said Grace, but when she became ill after three months she was returned to the Cascades Female Factory.

A fortnight later she 'was sent to a place where a shipmate lived whom I did not like so I told my mistress that I could not do "Housework"'. Back to Cascades. Her next assignment was miserable, 'I here wore all my clothes out and could not even obtain Soap to wash myself with. No money was given me—my food was Potatoes and Herrings and cakes made with ration flour bought from Prisoners in the Penitentiary'. Before long she 'ran away' but escaped 'punishment on stating my case to the Magistrate. A Lodger at this place asked me to prostitute myself to him, he was a married man and his wife selected me herself from the Factory. It was the ill treatment and abuse I received caused me to leave this place'.

After a week in the Female Factory, Grace was sent out to her fifth master in six months, and this time when she ran away she got into real trouble. She remained 'illegally at large' for a fortnight 'until apprehended by Constable Perkins last Evening in Company with a runaway Convict in a disorderly House in Watchorn Street'. She was punished by hard labour plus a six-month extension to her sentence.

The pattern was set— short periods of assignment, absconding, punishment. Even when she liked the household, she couldn't seem to settle, and spent much of her time inside the Female Factory. Her account is punctuated with stories of trafficking, of being able to get whatever you wanted as long as you had money. A turnkey sold bread for a shilling a loaf, a hospital nurse stole food from some prisoners, and sold to others. 'Those who have money can always get enough to eat whilst the others are Hungry.'

Superintendent Hutchinson appeared for muster each morning but the women 'did not see him afterwards unless there was a disturbance … The language used is very bad and fighting is common. There is no one present to check it'. One of Grace's punishments involved picking wool for about an hour each day, and then she and the other prisoners could 'sing, sew, run about and do anything to pass away the time. Some of the Women would act Plays, dress themselves up'. This was the heyday of the Flash Mob, and inside the massively overcrowded Female Factory, prisoners ran their own show.

Though Grace's account may have outraged the prison staff, it suited those members of the committee of enquiry who agreed with the mounting opinion that the Assignment System was open to abuse, and the female factories were dens of iniquity where reform played no role. Here was Grace, who had chalked up ten charges of absconding in four years, and showed no sign of mending her ways. Sentencing her to hard labour in the Female Factory could not be called a punishment. Extending her sentence (and her original seven-year sentence was now extended to eleven years) had no discernible effect—and yet, it may have made her susceptible to the bait offered for her story-telling. On 2 March 1842 Grace entered the Female Factory to serve a sentence of four months hard labour for absconding yet again. On 20 March her statement was taken down for the committee of inquiry. On 1 April she was recommended for a Conditional Pardon 'for the satisfactory manner' in which she gave her evidence. A prize-winning story!

ELIZA BENWELL

Eliza Benwell made a bad choice. Single and in her mid-thirties, she pawned property, including jewellery, stolen from the lodging house of her recently deceased mistress, Jane Coghlan who had left Eliza some things in her will, but Eliza could not wait. Living with Charles Wright as his wife, they had pawned the dead woman's goods at various establishments across London. When arrested Eliza claimed that her wages and inheritance remained unpaid. No one believed her defence, that her ailing mistress had told her to keep certain things and sell them for money if needed. Instead Wright was found not guilty, but Eliza was sentenced to two terms of seven years transportation for unlawfully pledging. This meant she would have to serve one full term and then four years of the second term before a Ticket of Leave could be granted by the Governor, rather than apply after only six years if given a fourteen year sentence.

On 13 June 1835 Eliza set sail on the *Hector* for Van Diemen's Land. She said she was a plain cook and house-maid and unlike many others who claimed these skills, she had worked in service. Her family remained in

Reading, Berkshire, but one brother, Charles, would join her in the colony.

At the time of the 1835 muster, Eliza was assigned to Captain Gardiner. A cook made a valuable addition to a colonial household and Eliza was relatively well behaved and only admonished once for being drunk in Gardiner's service, in 1837. Her next offence for drunkenness and being in a disorderly house resulted in a term of hard labour at the Cascades Female Factory. Her Ticket of Leave was suspended and she was only to be assigned in the Interior. Interestingly, Eliza gained her Ticket of Leave after only six years, regardless of the intent of the judge at the Central Criminal Court. In 1842 she returned to Cascades charged with immoral conduct and sentenced to the Second Class for hard labour. Eliza's third visit to Cascades and another term of hard labour occurred in 1845.

Early 1845, she was assigned to Mr Elwin of the Derwent Hotel, New Norfolk and employed as a housemaid. Other staff included Isaac Lockwood, a waiter, Thomas Gomm, the cook, and William Taylor, the ostler. Mr Hathaway, the American Consul, took his family to New Norfolk on holiday. With his family was Jane Saunders, a nursemaid, and Keo Moi Tiki, a young boy and servant from the Sandwich Islands (Hawaii). Late on the night of 18 January, Jane went missing. After a search, her body was found in the river a few metres from Elwin's jetty. Weston, the surgeon, determined she had died of suffocation before her body was disposed of in the water.

Isaac Lockwood was a suspect, having attempted to force his way into Jane's room. Apparently, Jane had threatened to report his behaviour to her master and have Lockwood sent to Port Arthur. Lockwood, Taylor and Gomm were arrested and charged with Jane's death. At the trial, the evidence of the young boy, Keo, was critical. Having watched the drama unfold from the upstairs window and also the garden, he testified for fourteen hours through an interpreter. He had seen Eliza talking with Jane in the garden, before the three men— Lockwood, Gomm and Taylor—assaulted Jane and suffocated her. They then moved her body to a boat. After half an hour the jury found the men guilty and sentenced them to death, following which their bodies were to be dissected. Eliza was to face a trial of her own.

Tried for aiding and abetting in the perpetration of the wilful murder of Jane Saunders, by suffocation, Eliza was sentenced to death on 11

September 1845. Insisting that Keo's evidence was false, she was afraid as Lockwood had forced her to take an oath, and threatened to kill her if she told anyone. She declared that she was prepared to meet her God.

Her fellow workmates, found guilty of the murder of Jane, were executed in front of the Hobart Gaol on 23 September 1845. Taylor went to his death stating that if Eliza Benwell and the two other men would tell all they knew they could save his life. After the bodies were cut down, they were taken to the Colonial Hospital and to St Mary's Hospital for dissection. This too would be Eliza's fate.

On 31 September at 8 am, Eliza climbed the scaffold to face Solomon Blay, her executioner and an ex-convict himself. One newspaper reported up to 5000 people gathered for the event, including many respectable women and children, especially boys. Eliza, dressed as for her trial, did not utter a word, conducting herself with decorum. When her body dropped many of the women screamed, others sobbed and wept. By 8.15, the crowd had dispersed. Reverend J. Therry submitted a statement from Eliza to the press, again pleading her case and stating her innocence.

The newspapers continued to report on Eliza's trial and execution. The editor of the *Hobart Town Advertiser* shared the horror of his observations in the dissecting room at the Colonial Hospital. When Eliza's body arrived, parts of Taylor's body remained on the dissecting table, a week after his execution. One paper reported that Eliza had confessed that she could have saved Jane had she known what was intended. Eliza said, too late, that Gomm and Taylor had no part in the murder and confirmed it was not premeditated.

The *Colonial Times* reported sympathetically on this 'unfortunate woman' and commented that when compared with other women of her class, she had only been before the police three times in ten years. This report was followed by the story of the jury members who had to pay for their own accommodation for the week of the trial. An indignity indeed!

Only two years later, on 14 September 1847, some 600 people watched another murderer climb the scaffold. While the executioner adjusted the rope and put the cap over his face, someone in the crowd would have whispered, 'He's her brother. That is Charles Benwell'.

MARY ANN CUMMINGS

Mary Ann Cummings' husband, recorded as Richard Cummins, was at sea aboard a man-of-war when his wife stood at the dock charged with stealing a blanket, shirt and quilt at Devonport, England in February 1848. Richard was probably a sailor with the British Royal Navy. Devonport, once named Plymouth Dock, and one of the largest naval establishments in the county, was a large town with a thriving ship building industry. Mary Ann's father and three brothers were alive when she was transported, but when she was charged she may have stood alone. She was 35 and childless. Her complexion was dark, her face long, eyes grey and she had black hair.

Mary Ann was skilled. She could read and write and she was a tailoress, who could not only sew but also cut out patterns, a skill that would prove useful aboard the *Tory* (3). She sailed from England in April 1848 with over 170 women and 13 children. The Surgeon Superintendent on board, Charles Smith, kept a detailed diary of the voyage. He was later the surgeon for the voyage on the *Duke of Cornwall* in 1850.

Dr Smith commented that the convict women on the *Tory* were 'generally thin and pale'. He attributed this to their time in prison awaiting transportation and he was aware of the depression many suffered at the thought of leaving friends and family behind. Many women experienced digestive problems early in the voyage, and constipation and headaches were common. When women presented with symptoms of hysteria, Dr Smith blamed the lives they had lived before conviction and the moral situation in which they found themselves. He tried to ensure cheerfulness on board by ensuring the women were occupied. He believed that constant employment was beneficial to health, comfort and happiness.

During the voyage the women sewed 500 shirts and knitted various items. Mary Ann may have taught some of her fellow convicts how to cut the patterns. Each morning and evening schools taught reading and writing and again, Mary Ann's skills may have been useful. Time was set aside each day for religious instruction and Dr Smith tried to encourage those women sinking into despondency by pointing out how they could do well in the colony. He promised great advantages could come to them if they followed a 'regular and industrious course of life'.

Routine was vital on board and each day the women aired bedding by hanging it in the riggings. Dr Smith insisted on personal cleanliness as well and made sure that underclothing was changed often. During the voyage the women lost that 'pale and sallow look' and by the time they were discharged to the hulk *Anson* in August 1850, all but four were in good health.

After serving her six months probation on the *Anson*, Mary Ann was discharged to the Brickfields Hiring Depot. In 1851 she was charged twice with drunkenness. Her only indulgence was a Ticket of Leave issued in September 1851. For Mary Ann the promised better life in the colony did not eventuate. In August 1852 she was found wandering about the town and taken to the Cascades Female Factory infirmary. She was 'quite mad'. Four weeks later she was dead.

An inquest held at Cascades on 15 September 1852 before Algernon Burdett Jones found that Mary Ann, still a prisoner, died of 'paralysis consequent on insanity'. Catherine White, the officer in charge of the hospital at Cascades, identified the body lying in the dead house as that of Mary Ann. Catherine told the inquest that Mary Ann was quite mad from the time she was placed in the hospital under observation. Mr Benson, the Medical Officer, saw her each day and swore she was given every comfort in hospital that could be afforded her. Mary Ann was violent and, at times, had to be restrained by force.

William Benson found Mary Ann of impaired intellect when she was admitted. No longer was she the skilled, literate woman who was sent to the colony. After he and the Principal Medical Officer discussed her case, she was declared insane with a recommendation for removal to the Lunatic Asylum at New Norfolk. Before her transfer could be organised, she suffered paralysis of her right side and lost her speech. After five days her speech returned, but her violence, delirious ravings and the odours from her bed became so offensive that she was moved from the infirmary to a separate apartment, normally a punishment cell, where she stayed until her death. Dr Benson reported that he knew nothing of Mary Ann's previous mental history.

Margaret Latham, a prisoner at Cascades, knew Mary Ann well. She had sailed on the *Tory* with her four years earlier. From that time, until she saw Mary Ann at Cascades she had not seen her at all, but was certain that the body in the dead house was Mary Ann Cummings. Mary McKenzie cared for her in the separate apartment. She and another woman sat with her overnight. Mary Ann had a good bed and plenty of clothing, every comfort she required, reported Margaret. When Mary Ann Cummings died a little after four o'clock in the morning of 13 September 1852 she did not die alone.

MARY

9

BRAID

Mary Braid and her brother Thomas were not the only siblings transported to Van Diemen's Land for incest and murder. English missionary John McKay and his sister Helen were tried in India for similar offences. What is different about the tale of Mary and Thomas is the very public and salacious manner in which their relationship was reported in the press. In the case of the McKays, the Indian press only hinted at the incestuous relationship and instead focussed on the masochistic murder of John McKay's daughter by her aunt. The Scottish press focussed on the very specific relationship between Mary and Thomas Braid, reporting on the incest between brother and sister 'german', an archaic term meaning full-sister rather than half-sister or step-sister. Broadsheets printed details of this 'crime against the laws of God'. The Scottish court punished Mary with a death sentence, yet only sentenced her brother to banishment. Helen McKay also received a harsher sentence than her brother.

Mary Braid was born in Liberton, Edinburgh in 1795, the eldest daughter of John Braid and Janet Begbie. She had five sisters and a brother.

Mary married Robert Morrison, a gentleman's servant and in 1822 they had a daughter, also named Mary. Robert died shortly after and Mary and her daughter returned to live at her mother's residence. This was a one-roomed apartment with two beds, one in which slept Mary with her daughter. It became very crowded once Mary's sister Helen and her 26-year-old brother Thomas returned home. Sometimes Mary slept next door at the Pringle's apartment, but this arrangement stopped after she had an argument with Euphemia Pringle with whom she shared a bed. This may have been to do with the fact that Mary and John Pringle, a widower, had a relationship. Perhaps Pringle had even offered to marry Mary, but Pringle's evidence during the trial in relation to this proposal was contradictory.

Thomas Braid was convicted of desertion and sentenced to seven years transportation in London in 1827. He received a Free Pardon and was discharged from the *Gangmede* hulk at Woolwich in May 1832. For this offence he never left England's shores. How pleased his family must have been to see him return to Edinburgh.

According to evidence given in court by 36 witnesses in a trial that lasted over 18 hours, between February 1832 and May 1833 Mary and Thomas Braid began an incestuous relationship in the family home. They then moved to a property belonging to Charity Anderson, a widow who rented out rooms, where they lived as husband and wife.

In April 1833 Mary gave birth to a girl. She later told the court that the child's father was John Loudie and that the accusation that her brother was father to the child was vindictive behaviour on the part of her sister, Ann, whose suggestions instigated the prosecution.

Around 16 August 1833 a rope was fastened around the neck of the baby and stones were attached to weigh her down after which she was thrown into the Edinburgh and Glasgow Union Canal. The body remained in the water for upwards of a week before she was discovered. Poor, young Mary Braid was only ten when she was required to identify the body of this child. She said she did not recognise it as the child she had seen with her mother. Mary's protestations that she was innocent of the child's murder fell on deaf ears and in February 1834 the court sentenced her to execution with her body to be buried within the prison walls, hence denying her a Christian burial in consecrated ground. Thomas was found guilty of incest, but not of murder.

While Mary languished in prison dangerously ill with typhus, Thomas was transported to Van Diemen's Land on board the *William Metcalfe* arriving in 1834. He was more forthright when stating his offence admitting 'I was also indicted for the murder of the child which I had by my sister'. The *Caledonian Mercury* of 15 February 1834 printed a report of Thomas's confession of the murder of the child in which he admitted to being the sole perpetrator. He said his sister knew nothing of it and was not an accessory. Mary's death sentence was commuted after a petition setting out the facts of Thomas's confession and signed by 150 people from the parish of Liberton. Instead, Mary was sentenced to transportation for Life. Initially there was some doubt that she would live long enough to know of the outcome of the petition for clemency. She had plenty of time to reflect on the fact that her infant child was poisoned by the baby's father who then threw the dead body into the canal.

Thomas's behaviour in Van Diemen's Land led to his imprisonment at Port Arthur. He exposed his person to a female infant resulting in fifty lashes and three years in chains. He served his time at Port Arthur, gained a Ticket of Leave in 1843 and later was mustered at Campbell Town.

In 1835 Mary arrived in Hobart on the *Hector*. Also on board was her 13-year-old daughter Mary, who was sent straight to the Queen's Orphan School. On board, the surgeon had reported Mary as 'remarkably well behaved'. She was highly skilled and with experience as a cook, housemaid and needlewoman, she was very employable. She went to work in the home of Dr Ross, who was most probably the editor of the *Hobart Town Courier*.

Mary was relatively well behaved in the colony, though in 1840 she was sent to the Cascades Female Factory for drunkenness and there spent 30 days in the cells. At this time she was working at Government House. While working for Sly in 1841 she was charged with neglect of duty and spent 14 days in the much harsher separate working cells. When she left the Factory Mary went to work for S.R. Dawson of Clarence Plains. This is probably Samuel Robinson Dawson who supervised the construction of St Matthew's Anglican Church at Rokeby.

We do not know if Mary and Thomas Braid saw each other in the colony, though we do know that the MacKays spent time together and that John was even a witness at his sister's wedding. Perhaps Thomas did not live long enough to see his sister, as he died in the service of Mr J.A. Winter in May 1844. His death was registered at Campbell Town, some distance from his sister in Hobart.

Mary gained her Conditional Pardon in 1846. Her daughter was returned to her care. Young Mary was discharged from the Orphan School in June 1856 to Dr Ross for whom her mother worked. Other than her crime, Mary was regarded as respectable and as a highly skilled servant. Perhaps she found her niche working for one of Hobart's more prominent citizens.

ELLEN BERCARY

10

Irish-born Ellen Bercary arrived in Hobart Town on the *Arabian* on 25 February 1847.

Ellen was tried in Tipperary in July 1846 and sentenced to transportation for Life, on her first conviction, for being an accessory to the murder of her husband of 25 years. She stated 'I am quite innocent of the charges' and claimed that her husband had three times been served with a notice to quit the place where they lived and when he refused, 'they came and killed him in bed by my side'. Despite her protestations, Ellen was found guilty.

Ellen, who was Roman Catholic and could read and write a little, was a 38-year-old country servant and dairy woman just over 5 feet 4 inches tall, with a sallow complexion, grey black hair, and hazel eyes. She had blue dots on the side of her nose. Her four brothers and two sisters were in Tipperary and her six children may have been with them.

Beginning her colonial career at the Brickfields Ellen was later assigned to various employers in Hobart. She was well behaved and had only one colonial offence—in April 1852 she was found guilty of being absent without leave and was sentenced to three months hard labour at the Cascades Female Factory. While in the Factory, she was sentenced to three days on bread and water for not performing her work. After this, Ellen remained out of trouble and was granted her Ticket of Leave in December 1854. A Conditional Pardon followed in November 1856.

Ellen and John Elford Hore applied for permission to marry in February 1853 and became husband and wife the following month, on 28 March, in St George's Church of England in Battery Point. John was a convict from Cornwall but had been tried in Devon. He arrived on the *Equestrian* (2) in October 1845, transported for stealing mahogany. When he was transported, John was married with five children. At the time of his marriage to Ellen, he was 42 and a sawyer.

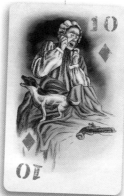

Ellen Hore died at Sale in Victoria on 1 January 1876.

At least one of Ellen's children followed her to Australia. Her son Jeremiah from her first marriage contested the granting of administration of her estate to her colonial husband, John Hore. Jeremiah claimed that a few days before she died, Ellen drew up a will in his favour. A protracted legal battle ensued.

ROSANNAH

Ⓙ MACDOWELL &

SARAH STANHOPE

When Rosannah MacDowell disembarked from the *Harmony* in January 1829, a gaol report came with her: 'has been trained up in the commission of crimes, her father, mother, brother, sisters and her two husbands have all been transported'. Rosannah herself proclaimed her criminal connections when asked to state her offence: 'My own father Snowden Dunning [or Dunhill] is here. George Dunning was my brother'. George had been hanged in Hobart Town on 3 July 1827 for stealing sheep. According to a local newspaper, George was 'aged 24, a handsome young man, about 6 feet 3 inches high, with a fine regular countenance'. His 'family and connections were numerous and most of them have been either executed or transported, having been long the dread of Yorkshire, noted as Snowden Dunhill's gang'.

Three months before the *Harmony* dropped anchor, Rosannah's half-sister Sarah Stanhope arrived on the *Borneo*. Her trial for what looks like a simple theft from a drunk had been reported extensively in the *Hull Packet* under the headline 'Trial of the Last of the Dunhills', and below the report was printed a biographical account headed 'Snowden Dunhill and his Family'. 'It is but rare in the history of crime', the account began, to find condensed 'into one family such an aggregate of guilt, and such a weight of judicial infliction'. When Sarah Stanhope was an infant, her own father had been shot and killed during an abortive robbery, and her mother had soon married Dunhill, a 'chief with a mysterious and unpleasant fame, such as might attach to the character of the *Rob Roy* of the East Riding'.

The matriarch of the gang was Snowden Dunhill's mother (and Rosannah MacDowell's grand-mother), whose first husband was hanged and her second transported. More than a decade before Rosannah and Sarah reached Hobart Town, the old woman stood at the bar in a York-shire courtroom, presenting 'some-thing of the grotesque and dreadful figure of *Meg Merrilies*'. Found guilty, 'she threw up her hands towards heaven, and hoped "*the Almighty would sink the whole Bench to perdition!*" In this profligate state she was taken back to the gaol, to undergo her future punishment, should her advanced age allow a continuance in life to undergo it'.

Sarah Stanhope and Rosannah MacDowell publically embraced their notorious connections, declaring for the colonial records their relationship to the legendary Dunhill. 'Snowden Dunhill married my mother', announced Sarah Stanhope. Given their high-profile criminal heritage, one might expect the members of this family to be nothing but trouble in Van Diemen's Land. And yet—with the early exception of brother George—this is not what happened.

Even the once-famous father of the clan dwindled to insignificance on the penal isle. The Rob Roy of Yorkshire became 'well known as a pieman about Hobart Town'. Perhaps in the hopes of reviving his highly publicised notoriety, he wrote (or more likely ghosted) an autobiography advertised for sale in his old stomping ground of Hull, but interest in the book proved short-lived, and when the name 'Snowden Dunhill' appeared in English newspapers, it soon referred to a racehorse running in the mid-century. The highwayman himself met an inglorious death in June 1838 as a prisoner at Port Arthur, described on the burial record as a labourer aged 76.

It may have taken Sarah Stanhope a little time to realise that notoriety in England would cut no ice in Van Diemen's Land. On the *Borneo* she courted the attention of the Surgeon Superintendent, determined to make a good impression on this man whose help she needed if she was to escape the rigours of the convict system by sailing with her two young daughters to Sydney. In Sydney she might be assigned to her transported husband, James Stanhope, alias 'One armed Jem', who was nearing the end of his sentence. Upon arrival in Hobart Town, the compliant Surgeon Superintendent duly supported her petition to the local Lieutenant-Governor, saying that throughout the voyage Sarah had behaved 'with great propriety'. Request denied. No special favours for criminal royalty from Home. Just as any other convict woman, Sarah would be sent out to work as an unpaid servant under surveillance.

Her ten-year-old daughter Rosanna may have gone with her, but eight-year-old Sarah Ann was confined in the Female Factory for four months before she and the other children from the *Borneo* were admitted into the King's Orphan School.

Only twice were charges entered on Sarah Stanhope's conduct record, and neither sent her back to the Female Factory. By the time of the second charge, for being drunk in 1832, she had been assigned to her now-free husband who had travelled from Sydney to reunite the family he scarcely knew. Sarah herself was free in January 1835, and seems to have died later that year.

Rosannah MacDowell was not quite as successful as Sarah in staying away from the new Cascades Female Factory. As a convict on the *Harmony* she was one of the first women sent there directly from the ship, and she too left behind a child when she was assigned. Her five-year-old son George spent ten months in the Nursery Yard before leaving for the Orphan School. Rosannah was back at Cascades in 1831, not for punishment but with a recommendation that she be assigned 'to the Interior' after she was charged with 'absenting herself from her service without leave, at the time she had her Master's child'. Somehow she talked her way out of the proposed banishment from town, and was back with the same master for the

1832 muster.

Meanwhile, her husband, Benjamin MacDowell, had also made his way to Hobart Town after he became Free by Servitude. The couple had spent scarcely any time together. They had married in April 1821, and in November that year Benjamin was on a convict transport bound for Sydney. The child Rosannah brought with her on the *Harmony* was not Benjamin's, which may explain why the little boy was left to grow up in the Orphan School while his mother started a new family with her husband.

Four children were born to this family who transformed themselves from a criminal gang in Yorkshire to farmers at Long Bay, now Middleton, on the D'Entrecasteaux Channel south of Hobart. There Rosannah MacDowell lived out the decades of her long life until she died 'of natural causes' on 27 May 1872, aged 75. As a widow whose farm was in her own name, she was a woman of property, and made a will to ensure that the division of assets accorded with her wishes. She divided the estate among the three surviving sons of Benjamin MacDowell, but because she had never learned to write her name, the signature 'in her sight and presence and by her direction' was that of her niece Sarah Ann, who sailed on the *Borneo* with her mother more than 40 years earlier. The descendants of the marauding Snowden Dunhill were now respectable citizens in Tasmania.

CHARLOTTE WILLIAMS

Charlotte Williams spoke no English and much of the court-proceeding at the Carmarthanshire Assizes would have sounded like gibberish to her. She did understand the witnesses giving testimony in her native Welsh, and she undoubtedly understood every word uttered by the prosecution's key witness, her 11-year-old daughter Rachel.

Charlotte's trial for sheep-stealing was high family drama. Here was a mother of nine children indicted along with three sons and two daughters, and according to Rachel, this mother was the mastermind of their trouble.

The Williams family were tenant farmers on the wind-swept slopes of the Black Mountain, one of the wildest parts of Wales. This was such a poor family that the children could not afford to marry, and even in their twenties remained at home. They may have had a cow or two, because there was a cow-house on the property, but mostly they relied on a few sheep to bring in cash. The father of the family, who was almost sixty, was already in gaol on a charge of stealing sheep from neighbours on the Black Mountain when Charlotte sent her sons up the same mountain to bring back their own sheep—and any others they might find.

When her sons came down with the sheep, her daughters helped separate their own animals from the others. After all the sheep were shorn, they killed the stolen sheep by knocking them on the head, and then took the wool into town to be sold. Unsurprisingly, the arrival of the Williams family with an unexpected quantity of wool aroused suspicion, and a warrant was issued to search the farm. On 23 June 1831 the searchers 'found the carcasses of 24 sheep buried in the ground near the cow-house, and 13 under a rock near the dwelling house'.

The trial of this sheep-stealing clan, according to a local newspaper, 'excited extreme interest in Court, on account of so many members of the same family being implicated in the crime; and of the extent of the depredations committed, but more particularly on account of its being necessary for the ends of justice to call a daughter of Charlotte Williams to bring home the charge to the prisoners'. Rachel, 'an interesting little girl about 11 years of age', was sternly examined by the judge before she gave her evidence. Could she read? he wanted to know, and could she say her prayers? 'No', came the reply to both questions. Well, did she know 'it was wicked to tell lies'? 'Yes', she said, she did. And did she know 'where people who tell lies went to after they were dead'? Yes, she said, they went to hell.

And then Rachel gave her damning testimony, an insider's account of her mother's inept plot. Rachel as the youngest child in this large family was suddenly asserting her place of power, and the others did not like it at all. In a courtroom where the prisoners were not represented by lawyers, they were allowed to ask questions of the witnesses, and the prisoners went on the attack. 'By whose directions' had Rachel come to swear her false testimony? She told them that she was there because David George asked her 'to say nothing but the truth'. And what had he promised her? they taunted, a new dress?

But of course, even if they had managed to discredit Rachel, the evidence spoke for itself, all those carcasses of dead sheep. Rachel's sisters escaped punishment on a legal technicality having to do with the wording of the indictment, but her older brothers Thomas and James were sentenced to transportation for Life, while mother Charlotte and her closest brother Evan (who was only 13) were sentenced to transportation for fourteen years.

The quirky story of a criminal family in the mountains of Wales made good copy for the press. 'A Family of Sheep-Stealers', read the headline for filler pieces picked up by newspapers in Ireland and England, even making it into the *Morning Post* of London. The effect on the actual family was traumatic.

Two of Charlotte's sons, 26-year-old Thomas and his youngest brother Evan sailed from London on the *Katherine Stewart Forbes* in February 1832, reaching Hobart on 16 July. Less than a year later, Thomas died in the Colonial Hospital. He may have been allowed a visit from his mother, recently arrived on the *Frances Charlotte*. Meanwhile, James, the oldest son, for some reason had been separated from his brothers (perhaps he too had been ill?), and when Thomas died, James had not yet sailed on the *Heroine*, which would take him to New South Wales.

Charlotte's husband would never actually be transported, living out his last days in a prison hulk moored in the River Thames. On 2 March 1835, two days before James Thomas Williams was buried in the London borough of Islington, the first and only charge against Charlotte Williams was entered on her conduct record.

The master to whom she was assigned charged her with neglect of duty, and she was reprimanded by the Principal Superintendent of Convicts in Van Diemen's Land, where she was serving out her sentence as a model convict, gaining a Conditional Pardon on 18 November 1841.

JULIA, ELIZABETH & EMILY SALT

The three sisters Salt—Julia Mary, Elizabeth Ann and Emily—were born in Cripplegate, London, and baptised in the nearby St Giles-without-Cripplegate church, one of the few remaining medieval churches in London to this day.

Julia, Mary and Emily were aged between ten and sixteen when the 1841 census passed through Royal Oak Walk, Hoxton Old Town, Shoreditch in Middlesex, England. The girls resided there with their father Thomas and mother Sarah, as well as two brothers, William and Thomas. Thomas Snr had listed three different professions on the baptism papers for his daughters: porter, plasterer and bricklayer. On the baptism records for William and Thomas, he was listed as 'labourer'. Perhaps a clue as to what influenced Thomas' daughters to pack up and move to the other side of the world and gain employment as warders in a Female House of Correction lies in his listed professions, or perhaps a calling influenced by their surroundings as children?

One of the roles Thomas lists is as a porter. With the actual 'gate' of London Wall's Cripplegate having been demolished in the 1760s, one of the more likely locales requiring a porter in the nearby area was the Debtors Prison or Whitecross Street Prison. Built in 1813 by the City of London, the prison was for the exclusive reception of debtors. Were the Salt sisters to become second generation prison employees, following in their father's footsteps? Perhaps it was simply the influence of their faith and veneration for St Giles—the patron of beggars, outcasts and poor people among others—that drove them to want to contribute to the reformation of female prisoners.

Regardless of their motivation, nine years after the census, the three girls were logged as steerage passengers on board the barque *Calcutta*, departing from London on 13 July 1850 bound for Hobart Town, Van Diemen's Land. They arrived with only 10 other passengers and 25 crew on 1 October. What the sisters got up to between disembarking and 1853 is difficult to establish, but perhaps an advertisement in the *Cornwall Chronicle* on 22 September 1852 caught their eye: 'A female warder is called for, at the Cascades Factory—salary £57 per annum, with quarters'.

Between September 1853 and December 1855 all three sisters had taken positions as warders within the Cascades Female Factory. The position of warder within the walls of the House of Correction would not have been an easy task, and had quite an imposition on the private life of those in the role.

Regulations of the Probationary Establishment for Female Convicts in Van Diemen's Land, 1 July 1845 … Assistants, Teachers, Warders and other Officers.

38. The assistants, teachers, warders and other officers will strictly conform to the rules of the establishment, obey the directions of the superintendent and matron, and zealously assist them in maintaining order and discipline. They are not to be absent without leave from the superintendent, and then only during the day, and never for more than four hours …

40. Written reports will be made by the assistants and warders daily in a report book, with which they are all to be provided, on such subjects as may be necessary to be brought under the notice of the superintendent, more particularly as regards the conduct of the women immediately under their charge.

How long the sisters stayed in the employ of the House of Correction is not 100 per cent clear, but Emily had returned to England prior to July 1855. Perhaps she had returned home due to the death of her father in October 1854. She came back to Hobart on the barque *Elizabeth* on 18 November 1855 with eighteen other passengers. Again travelling in steerage, Emily's five month journey would certainly not have been as comfortable as those passengers with a cabin, one of whom was listed as Mr Roderick Reynolds.

Emily took her role at the Female Factory just weeks after returning from England on 4 December, possibly taking a position her sister Elizabeth had vacated. Whether she and Roderick knew each other prior to their journey on the same ship from London is unknown, but something definitely brought this prison warder and school master together. Emily and Roderick were married in St Joseph's Church in Hobart on 30 May 1857. Not long after their marriage, Roderick was listed as a school master in Richmond and the first of their five children was born there. The family moved to Black Brush prior to 1863 when Roderick junior was born. This locale is also where Emily's life was cut short at the young age of just 35 on 6 October 1868.

Less is known about Julia, with the exception that less than a year after Emily wed so too did Julia, to James William Stuart in Hobart on 6 April 1858. James was 42, Julia ten years his junior. Julia passed away in her home at 136 Murray Street, Hobart on 18 June 1873 aged 47.

As for Elizabeth, the middle sister, her untimely death from fever while sub-matron of the Lunatic Asylum, was recorded in New Norfolk on 13 May 1860. The registration states she was only 24—but if the 1841 census for Middlesex was correct, she may well have been 31.

ISABELLA
BOSWELL

Isabella Boswell claimed to be 44 years of age when she arrived in Van Diemen's Land on board the *Aurora* (2) on 10 August 1851. Dr W.S.B. Jones described Isabella's behaviour during the journey as exemplary. She declared herself married, but a widow of nineteen years with two children. Tried at the Edinburgh Court of Justiciary for theft, Isabella was transported for seven years. She had stolen bacon from Mr Peters of Potter Row, Edinburgh and admitted that she had been convicted three times before, including stealing money and pawning a gown that presumably didn't belong to her. Isabella was a midwife, standing 5 feet 1¼ inches tall with black hair and hazel eyes, her face was slightly pockmarked.

Records in Scotland show that one Isabella Boswell married Alexander Nimmo on 1 March 1819 at Canongate, Edinburgh, Midlothian, Scotland, which would make Isabella only twelve at the time! Further records show that an Isabella Boswell was born to George and Janet Boswell in 1803 in Abercorn, West Lothian, Scotland, which if aligned with the marriage records, would make Isabella sixteen at the time of her marriage—if in fact they are the same person.

Eight days after disembarking from the ship, Isabella found herself at the Brickfields Hiring Depot, and shortly after assigned to T.S. Downie of Kelly Street, Battery Point. In early 1852 she was working for Mr Lovett in Davey Street, Hobart. On 21 February 1852 she appeared in the Female House of Correction, as a result of being charged with being drunk, and sentenced to two months hard labour. This behaviour was obviously not as common place for Isabella as a number of her peers, as she made her way up through the ranks quicker than usual to become a watchwoman.

Reporting on management of the Factory during January 1852, Superintendent James May described the role of the watchwoman and one of the small graces they received on account of their good behaviour:

The women composing the watch are those under sentence, who are invariably selected after two thirds of such a sentence have been performed in ordinary labour, and on account of their good and exemplary conduct. Every consistent encouragement being extended to them, their duties are generally faithfully performed. They are distinguished by their dress from the other prisoners in the establishment; this consists of a straw bonnet, blue serge jacket, and cotton gown, which impart to them a neat and uniform appearance.

Different clothes may seem like a small reprieve. However, every little permissible variation on the usually bleak convict uniform would have been gratefully received.

Superintendent May went on to describe the duties carried out by the watchwomen in the establishment:

During the day they assist the officers in carrying out the details of discipline of the establishment, and during the night a watchwoman is placed in each of the sleeping apartments, whose duty consists in perambulating the wards in which she is posted, keeping the lights brightly burning, and seeing that none of the regulations are in any particular infringed upon by the prisoners.

Unfortunately, being a watchwoman did not put you above the rules. On 23 March 1852 Mr Sidney, the Overseer of Weavers at the Factory, reported Isabella for neglect of duty as a watchwoman, her punishment being three days on bread and water.

Just over two months after neglecting her duty, on 29 May 1852, Isabella died at the Cascades Female Factory. The cause was listed as paralysis of the right side supervening on diarrhoea. Is it possible that Isabella died of a stroke?

In Superintendent May's report dated 10 July 1852, just weeks after the death of Isabella, he wrote—'The mortality amongst adults confined within the establishment during the last six months is considerably lower than that of the previous half year, three deaths only having taken place, being a decrease of two-thirds'.

Although the fewer deaths during the reporting period may have been seen as an achievement in the eyes of convict department, it is hard to imagine what Isabella's children back in Scotland would have felt hearing of their mother's passing on the opposite side of the world. That is, if they ever got the news.

SARAH
HUGHES

Sarah Hughes was 21 years old when she was brought before the judge at the Assizes at Taunton on 31 March 1846, having been accused of administering poison (sulphuric of copper) with intent to murder her infant child. Her sentence—death. A week later the sentencing judge wrote a letter petitioning for her sentence to be commuted to transportation for Life on the grounds that the jury and prosecution had strongly recommended that mercy be shown to Sarah. Furthermore, on 14 May 1846, another application for leniency was presented by Mr Dickinson MP while Sarah was being held in Millbank Prison. It included recognition of her background from the Reverend of the Doulting Parish in Somerset:

... [she] was left an orphan at a very early age, without brother, sister or any friend to guide or control her ... was led astray under the usual promise of marriage, as is alleged, whilst she was in farm service, and being driven from house and home, took refuge in the Union House of the district where in a fit of desparation [sic] she was tempted to commit the crime of which she was convicted; that during the time she was an inmate of the Shepton Mallet Gaol viz—five or six months—and subsequently, in Taunton Gaol, the Governors and Matrons of these gaols are ready to testify that she treated her child with the greatest tenderness and care, and that her behaviour, generally, was marked by a very unusual degree of propriety and decorum.

Sarah received a reprieve from execution, and on 21 September 1846 departed London on board the *Elizabeth & Henry* (2) with 169 other female convicts bound for Hobart.

On a voyage taking 109 days she was described as well behaved on board. Arriving on 4 January 1847, details recorded state that she was 5 feet 1 inch in height, with a very low forehead, a wide mouth and light brown hair, a country servant with dairy experience, she could also read. Though the petition declared she was without siblings, her record in Van Diemen's Land states she had a sister Mary at the time of transportation.

As with many of her contemporaries, Sarah was ordered on arrival to serve six months probation on the prison hulk *Anson* moored in Prince of Wales Bay on the Derwent River near Hobart. No offences were committed in the months after her arrival, but by November 1848 Sarah was at the Female Factory in Hobart and gave birth to an illegitimate child, Frederick. In December 1849, while Frederick was most likely in care at the Female Factory or the Dynnyrne Nursery, Sarah was in assigned service. However, due to poor behaviour was not allowed to enter service in Hobart. This arose from an attempt to abscond from service by removing her clothes from the house and concealing them under some bushes. Was she attempting to abscond so as to reconnect with her son? We will never know. Nor do we know whether she ever saw Frederick again. Sarah was in assigned service when she committed her second offence on 8 June 1850, this time stealing a blanket for which she was sentenced to 18 months hard labour at the Female Factory. Four days before this offence was committed Frederick died of acute dysentery at the Brickfields Hiring Depot for women—he was only 18 months old.

Assigned women were more in demand if unencumbered by children or pregnancy, but liaisons often occurred in hired service, and this may well have been what happened to Sarah for a second time. On 3 March 1852 she gave birth to another child who only survived five days. To add to her emotional burden, three weeks later she was charged with concealing the pregnancy and giving birth to an illegitimate child for which she received a cruel sentence—9 months hard labour!

Returning to the Factory, an additional note on her record states that she was to serve 15 months there from 12 June 1852, but by May 1853 Sarah relocated to the Female Factory at Ross, 120 kilometres north of Hobart. The Ross Factory was formerly a probation station for male convicts, and converted into a female hiring depot in 1848 to service the Midlands region. Sarah was in and out of the Ross Factory to assigned service in the area for the next three years before returning to Hobart and gaining a Ticket of Leave in December 1855. Now able to work for wages, no further offences were committed, and in February 1857 Sarah was recommended for a Conditional Pardon, which she gained on 29 September that year—10 years after her initial conviction.

It seems that during her time within the convict system Sarah Hughes did not make an application for permission to marry, and no subsequent marriage can be found. The birth of a child, Richard, to a Sarah Hughes and registered in Campbell Town on 12 June 1854 cannot be confirmed as Sarah's—though she was in the region at the time. Richard appears to have died in Hobart 14 months later, of diarrhoea. Whether Sarah had a total of 3 or 4 children, her experience with each was touched by sadness. Her fate is unknown.

SUSANNA

WEBB

Susanna Webb arrived on the *Arab* (3) in the autumn of 1836 with her babe in arms. Her husband, Charles,

remained at Sheldon. Susanna, a cook and house servant aged 28, had stolen tea and sugar from her master. Within weeks of arrival, her young son, also named Charles, died at the Cascades Factory. He was only nine months old.

Susanna was charged with insolence just two weeks after the death of her son. She spent ten days in a cell on bread and water. Later that year she claimed she was too ill to work, and she was detained to be examined by the surgeon. She had several other charges of absence without leave, insolence, disorderly conduct and threatening to leave her master's residence. She was well known at Cascades by the time she gained her Free Certificate in 1842.

John Ray and George Banning both applied to marry Susanna. After an ecclesiastical opinion was sought John Ray's petition was approved, but Susanna chose George Banning and the couple married at Holy Trinity in January 1840. She said she was 33 and a widow. He claimed to be 34 and a widower. George was a convict and had arrived in 1830 on the *Clyde*. He left a wife and two children in England. In 1851 Susanna and her husband sued for the false imprisonment of Susanna after she was wrongly taken into custody while George was imprisoned at Richmond for the non-payment of a crown fine. These were not people to mess with! In 1855

George Banning became proprietor of the Blue Bells of Scotland public house in Murray Street, Hobart.

George left the colony several times during the early 1850s, perhaps taking off for the goldfields and Susanna followed her husband to Melbourne in October 1852. Although on departure she told the authorities that she was born in the colonies, they noted that she was 'possibly Susannah Webb arriving aboard Arab'.

In 1859, *The Courier* reprinted an article from the *London Prototype and Daily Western Advocate* (Canada) about a sensational case of bigamy. George Banning was charged with incest, bigamy and being an escaped convict from Tasmania. Neither this paper, nor the *Birmingham Daily Post* mentioned that Susanna had also been a convict.

They reported Susanna's evidence about the legitimacy of her marriage in 1840 and her story after she left the colony. She said that when she married she was a servant with £100 to her name. She said that they had lived at Prosser's Bay in Tasmania for about ten years, and then they had moved to Melbourne, spending over two years there. George went to the goldfields and later opened a successful store in Melbourne. The couple was wealthy having about £30,000 pounds in ready money. They returned to Tasmania, purchased a farm at Prosser's Bay, but sold it shortly after and went to Sydney, before sailing for London.

They arrived in London in February 1857 and George immediately abandoned Susanna. It took her a couple of days to find him, in the company of a woman he claimed to be his sister. George denied being married to Susanna. Not to be trifled with, Susanna took him before a magistrate and produced her marriage certificate. George promised to treat her better and to provide for her. Less than a week later, on the train to Birmingham, he threatened to blow her brains out with a pistol and took away the marriage certificate, her wedding ring and other jewellery.

After another reconciliation they opened a tavern in Birmingham in Susanna's name as George had been transported for Life—although he had a Ticket of Leave and a Conditional Pardon for the Australian Colonies, neither enabled him to live in England nor take out a licence in his name. He could face being sent back to Australia if he was discovered. Susanna's Free Certificate meant that she was not regarded as an escaped convict.

The couple moved in with George's sister and brother-in-law. Susanna was treated badly, and was soon deserted by George who went to Canada, after an apparent incestuous relationship with his sister. While in Van Diemen's Land, Susanna had adopted a child, known as Mary Ann Banning, apparently the illegitimate child of an Australian connection who provided money for the child's upkeep. Susanna and Mary Ann, now aged about 17, tracked George to London, Ontario in Canada. Susanna was a determined woman. Did she want her husband back, or the £30,000 pounds he had left the country with?

In Canada, George had purchased a farm and was loaning money to those who could pay good interest. George's sisters appeared in court on his behalf and described Susanna as a 'drunken and violent woman'. One also admitted sleeping in the same bed as her brother and his wife, but denied the charge of incest. A newspaper advertisement from the *Birmingham Daily Post* of 13 April 1857 was admitted as evidence. In it, George warned the public not to trust his wife, 'Susanna Banning, alias Webb, alias Bishop, and alias Vale'.

The magistrates admitted George to bail, but later decided that there was insufficient evidence and discharged him. Susanna must have been furious. The money was gone, but she still had the tavern, as it was in her name! She returned to Birmingham to her public house the Wharf Tavern, Wharf Street. In the 1858 edition of *Dix's General and Commercial Directory of Birmingham* Susannah Banning of 2 Oosells Street was listed as a retail brewer.

Mary ♠ Pullen

The fifth session of the Old Bailey proceedings was held at Justice Hall on Thursday 29 May 1828. In one of many trials on the day, Mary Pullen was brought before the magistrate for stealing on 20 February two tablecloths, value 6 shillings, and one flat iron, value 1 shilling, the property of publican William Dyas, of North Audley Street. Mary had been employed as a washerwoman by William, who noticed that his aforementioned property was missing. Following evidence from two other women, a pawnbroker and an officer, Mary was found guilty of the crime and sentenced to be transported for seven years. She was 27.

At the time, her father Thomas was gardener to the Governor of Windsor, Charles Stanhope, and 3rd Earl of Harrington, a former soldier and retired Commander-in-Chief in Ireland. It was unlikely she would ever see her father and mother, Mary, again after boarding the *Harmony* and departing Downs in southern England in September 1828 for Van Diemen's Land. The voyage took 123 days, and carried 63 passengers including 8 free women and 33 children. Ten weeks into the voyage, Mary suffered with *menorrhagia* (heavy or prolonged menstrual bleeding) for 12 days. However, she recovered and on 14 January 1829 the ship arrived in Hobart—all 100 female convicts on board had survived.

Lieutenant-Governor George Arthur desired that all convict ships berthed in Hobart so as to secure the collection of information gathered about the convicts, by recording it in one place. The Muster Master's role was to maintain the records containing the details on the convicts and he boarded the ships to record their description, details of former life, transportation crime and sentence, and previous convictions. Mary was described as a plain cook and laundry maid, 5 feet 3 inches in height, with features including a sharp pointed nose, perpendicular forehead, oval visage and high temples, brown hair and a fair complexion.

As Mary arrived during the Assign-ment Period of convict administration, convict men and women were generally allocated to work for a free settler on arrival. Mary was in the service of the Reverend William Bedford, who had been Minister of St David's Church for almost 30 years. On 16 April 1829, barely three months after arriving, she was found drunk and disorderly and in bed with one of his male servants. For this she was relegated to Crime Class status at the Female House of Correction or Female Factory in Hobart, and in a cell on bread and water for seven days.

By the end of December of that same year she was assigned to Miss Steele and again returned to the Female Factory 'until further orders' for drunkenness and suspicion of having stolen articles of Miss Steele's property. Her period of detention is unknown, and Mary is otherwise well behaved—until January 1831.

Now in the service of Mr Commissary Brown, drunkenness reared its head again for Mary and she was found 'harbouring a strange man in her master's house'. The Crime Class at the Female Factory was again her punishment—hard labour, and confinement in a cell on bread and water for six days. She was returned to Brown, but in August of the same year her weakness for alcohol brought about another sentence of seven days confinement on bread and water. This was Mary's last recorded offence.

All four colonial offences included reference to alcohol. At the time, societal standards did not deem it appropriate for a woman to indulge to the extent that it led to drunkenness. It was a common offence of convict women and they were penalised for it. Governor of New South Wales, George Gipps, stated a few years later in 1841, 'there is nothing in the whole catalogue of crime, so thoroughly revolting as drunkedness in a woman; there is no object of disgust or horror that offends the sight of God or man, so entirely as a drunken woman'.

Whatever led to Mary's desire or weakness for alcohol, no further offences were committed after August 1831. She was 30 years of age. No application was made by her for permission to marry anyone, and no marriage, birth or death references have been found.

The *Hobart Town Courier* of Friday 1 May 1835 printed a Government notice from the Colonial Secretary's Office stating that those whose names were listed, could obtain a Certificate of Freedom, their period of transportation having expired. The certificates could be obtained 'then, or at any subsequent period, upon application at the Muster Master's office,

Hobart Town, or at that of a Police Magistrate in the interior'. Mary's name was listed among a number of her fellow prisoners who had arrived in Hobart on the *Harmony* over six years earlier.

Whether she collected her Certificate we will never know and her fate is equally obscure but she may have left Van Diemen's Land. A Mary Pullen departed on the *Perseverance* as a passenger in early January 1840, leaving from George Town for Port Phillip—perhaps for a better life?

♠5 ELIZA MCINTYRE

Dear Eliza, dear Eliza. Eliza McIntyre was 'repeatedly imprisoned as a disorderly character'. Recorded as having been imprisoned some twenty times prior to her transportation, it appears that Eliza had a fervent habit of acquiring goods that didn't belong to her and a weakness for an ale or two. A far stretch from the perception of a poor young girl transported for stealing a handkerchief, it was a watch belonging to Mr Edward Rouse that was Eliza's undoing.

A 32-year-old laundress hailing from Marylebone, Eliza was convicted on the same day as Charles McIntyre, twelve years her junior—whether they were related or not is unknown, but

Eliza only listed a brother George and sister Anne as her relatives. With the theft of the watch being the final straw, Eliza was sentenced to ten years transportation and loaded aboard the *Lloyds* with 170 other women bound for Van Diemen's Land. Her relationship with Thomas Norman is also a mystery but Eliza listed him as the individual she had lived with for the six years prior to her transportation.

Despite her reputation, the surgeon on board the *Lloyds* reported that Eliza was very well behaved and industrious and that he would recommend her. Perhaps when the ship docked in Hobart Town in November 1845, Eliza was keen to start afresh as it appears that for her first six months in the colony, she stuck to the rules. It was a charge of misconduct and being out after hours in July and September of 1846 that appear to have diverted Eliza from her new found path of good behaviour.

During the next eight years some twenty crimes were recorded on Eliza's conduct record, many of which could be put down to 'getting lost' on the way to and from work. Unfortunately for Eliza, that plea is harder to sell to the authorities with alcohol on your breath. Being absent or drunk resulted in sentences total-ing over four years of hard labour. A large proportion of her hard labour sentences were carried out at the Cascades Female Factory, more than likely in Yard 2 of the establishment.

Hard labour was usually directed towards washing—laundering for both the convict establishment and the free settlers of the colony. During the mid-1800s Hobart's free used the institution much as we use a laundromat or dry cleaners today. Despite Eliza's trade being documented as laundress, it would appear that on occasion Eliza dreamed of a different life, resulting in neglect of duty being noted on her record on more than one occasion.

Despite the many blemishes on her record, Eliza's sentence was not lengthened and she received her freedom after her ten year sentence had expired, and although it is impossible to be certain if it is the same Eliza McIntyre, one appears in the *Hobart Town Daily Mercury's* Police Report in late 1855, early 1858 and mid-1859. Initially reported as a 'drunkard' and fined 20 shillings, this 'very old offender and frequenter of the watch-house' was also charged with being a common prostitute and sentenced to one months imprisonment. A later charge for being an 'idle and disorderly character, in being found sleeping in the open air and having no visible means of subsistence' resulted in three months imprisonment. If this was our dear Eliza, by 1859 she was in her mid-40s and perhaps finally ready for that different life.

Eliza disappeared from the Police Court pages of the newspaper and little else would be known about her except for the occasion of an enquiry as to her whereabouts made by Hobart law firm Giblin & Dobson in June 1866. Either a guilty conscience or perhaps genuine fear caused Eliza to respond in writing to the government stating her location and requesting a response as to the purpose of the enquiry.

Dear Sir

Having seen your inquiry for me in your Gazette I write to inform you I am Eliza McIntyre by the Lloyds free in 1855 and should be glad if you will condesend to return me a answer as to the reason of the Enquiry as I have been in the greatest anxiety this six months from enquirys made from England to Mssr Gibling & Dobson and can git no information from who as why the inquirys are made. I trust you will condesend to relieve my unhappy mind if you can as I have never heard Direct from those belonging to me since I have been from England but had many inquirys a few years back from your office. I remain your humble servant

Eliza McIntyre
Direct from me
Oatlands Post Office

Perhaps Thomas Norman had tried to find Eliza, or her family from England? Either way, it appears Eliza was happy in Oatlands and perhaps just wanted to be left alone.

ELIZABETH
MACK

On 31 March 1849 the biannual Assize Court for the North and South Wales Circuit, which included the county of Cheshire, held a sitting in Chester. It was led by an itinerant judge, typical of the Assizes. Elizabeth Mack, a housemaid and married woman from Manchester, was tried for receiving stolen goods. With Finnie stated as her proper name, her husband John was tried with her for the same offence. Having been found guilty, she was sentenced to ten years and transportation across the sea, leaving behind two children, a brother John, and sister, Sarah. There is no evidence that her husband was transported.

The penultimate voyage of the *St Vincent* (I) as a convict ship to Hobart departed London in December 1849, carrying 205 female convicts under the captaincy of John Young. Its next voyage, arriving in May 1853, was the last ship carrying convicts to Van Diemen's Land—closing the transportation chapter of Tasmania's history. Elizabeth was on board when it docked in Hobart on 4 April 1850. As with all other convicts, her physical characteristics and background details were recorded: 35 years of age, a native of Manchester, Protestant and able to read, 5 feet 3 inches in height, with a pale complexion, long head, dark brown hair, light hazel eyes and a high forehead.

Assigned on arrival to a free settler, she experienced her first taste of the Female Factory in Hobart in early August 1851 when, in the service of her master, Bilton, she was found to have a man secreted in her bedroom. Such dalliances were frowned upon and an irritation for employers of female servants—concealment as Elizabeth attempted, was common. She didn't end up in 'the family way', the term used by Lieutenant-Governor Arthur some years earlier in complaining about similar behaviour, but she was removed from her service to experience six months hard labour, probably to the frustration of her master.

Following their stint in confinement, female convicts would again be hired out to assigned service, often via the Brickfields Hiring Depot in New Town—Elizabeth was there on New Year's Day 1852. The next day she was assigned to a residence in New Town Road for two weeks, then back to Brickfields for two days. Out to service again in the city of Hobart for eleven days, back to Brickfields for six days, and then out again. This routine was repeated until March 1852 when she absconded from C. Callaghan in Goulburn Street, Hobart. Her punishment was six months hard labour at the Female Factory.

About six weeks later, Elizabeth was to again experience solitary confinement. Those sentenced to hard labour, as she had been previously, were subjected to 'separate treatment' for the first half of their sentence. On this occasion, the sentence for the Factory offence of 'having a quantity of tea in the cookhouse for which she could not satisfactorily account' led to the short sentence of three days solitary. This was typical for such breaches of regulations. Elizabeth was also to be kept at the wash tub, her work credits stopped and she was not again to be employed in any billet. The regulations approved by the Lieutenant-Governor in 1851 included that every prisoner in solitary confinement must be strictly searched and all articles taken away, no communications were to take place with other prisoners, perfect cleanliness was essential, and four yards distance was to be kept between prisoners when out of their cells for exercise for no more than an hour a day—half an hour in the morning and the remainder in the afternoon. Yard 2 was the location of the 'wash tub' where clothes and linen were laundered by hand. Items washed included family clothing, blankets, palliasses (thin straw-filled mattresses), rugs, sheets, slop shirts, and hospital clothing. It was hard work and the women were subject to the vagaries of the weather.

Despite the reference that Elizabeth not be employed in any billet, by August 1852 she was in service again to B.C. Johnson at Kangaroo Point (now Bellerive). It is not known how long she worked there, but she was fined 5 shillings for using indecent language in August 1853, then removed to the Female Factory again for the same offence in January 1854—this time the magistrate sentenced her to one month hard labour.

The following month Elizabeth relocated to work at the Turnbull residence at New Norfolk, 38 kilometres west of Hobart, and in November to the family of Charles Maddox of Macquarie Plains, approximately 17 kilometres west of New Norfolk. Charles and his wife, Susan, had three children at the time. Elizabeth remained in their service until March 1855 when she returned to New Norfolk to the service of E. Terry.

It may have been while in the service of Charles Maddox that Elizabeth met her future husband, William Beanes. They had applied for permission to marry in January 1855, but it was noted that approval would only be given if she was free of offence for six months. On fulfilling that requirement, approval was given on 6 June 1855, and they married at St Mary's Church, Macquarie Plains on 5 July. The marriage registration described Elizabeth as a widow, and William a labourer, and her former master Charles Maddox appeared as a witness to the event.

Elizabeth had now been in the colony five years. On 12 February 1856 she was granted a Ticket of Leave, allowing her to work for wages and by October was recommended for a Conditional Pardon, which was granted in June 1857. She committed no further offences. As was typical of most female convicts in Van Diemen's Land, she had experienced the confines and hard labour at a female convict institution, as well as assigned service, but the remainder of her life is a mystery—no apparent births or death, no census or departure references could be found, and her former life in England no more than a distant memory.

BIDDY YACK McKENNA

Biddy Yack McKenna, described as 'infamous' in her Irish gaol report, was tried in Tyrone in Ireland on 2 July 1844 for stealing from the person. Unusually, she was sentenced to transportation for seven years—twice (on two indictments).

Arriving on the *Phoebe* on 2 January 1845, she stated her offence to be stealing a turkey from the person and also an apron. She had two previous convictions, both for assault, and had been brought before the court several times for drunkenness, a practice she unfortunately continued in Van Diemen's Land.

Biddy, aged 36, was a housemaid from Tyrone, with a fair complexion, brown hair, grey eyes and a round dimpled chin. Her straight nose was scarred. 'Scar corner of nose left side.' She was Roman Catholic and illiterate, characteristics shared with many of the Irish convict women. There was some confusion about Biddy's marital status—perhaps she was on the look-out for a colonial husband because she was recorded as both married and single! She claimed that she had been married by a drunken clergyman and she did not consider it a legal marriage—'we

were all drunk'. However, she lived with that 'husband' for four years. In December 1854 Biddy's application to marry fellow convict Henry Smith, who had arrived on the *Elphinstone*, was conditionally approved, if the clergyman agreed, but the marriage does not seem to have gone ahead.

Biddy's first recorded colonial offence was on 14 January 1847 when she was sentenced to one month hard labour at the Cascades Female Factory for misconduct and being drunk. From this time, Biddy was a regular inhabitant of the Factory. In August 1847 she was charged with drunkenness, using obscene language and assaulting a constable. For this, she was sent to the Factory for four months with hard labour—but she did not learn from the experience and was sent to the Factory again in March 1848, to serve a three month sentence with hard labour for being absent. Again, in September 1848, she was found absent without leave and received one month hard labour and in July 1849 Biddy was sentenced to another three months hard labour for being absent without leave and refusing to work. As far as Biddy was concerned, it seems that rules were made to be broken!

In November 1849, at the Brickfields, Biddy was accused of being drunk—yet again—and was sent to the Factory for another three month spell with hard labour. She was twice charged with the more serious offence of absconding in 1849.

On 23 April 1850, in private service, she was charged with being drunk and was sentenced to six months hard labour at the Cascades Female Factory and was 'Not to be allowed to enter service in the District of Hobart Town'. In March 1851 she was guilty of being out after hours and earned another month in the Factory. Later that year, in September, and again in February 1852, she was sent to the Factory— in September, she was sentenced to four months imprisonment with hard labour for being absent without leave and drunk, in February she received a much more severe sentence of eight months imprisonment with hard labour. It was ordered yet again that she not be allowed to enter service in the District of Hobart Town. In November 1852, in private service, Biddy was charged with being drunk and out after hours. This time she was sent to the Factory for eight months imprisonment with hard labour. In October 1853, she was drunk and out after hours, and received another sentence of four months imprisonment with hard labour. She was clearly not a model servant.

By December 1854, Biddy had gained her Ticket of Leave but she continued to be charged with drink-related offences, including disturbing the peace—from December 1854 to July 1858, she was charged eight times. Her punishment included seven days solitary confinement, fourteen days solitary confinement, one month hard labour, three months hard labour (three times). During this time she absconded in August 1856 and a reward of ten shillings was offered for her apprehension, which was successful late the following month. Then in April 1857 while working in the hospital she received five days hard labour for disturbing the peace.

Having served her two sentences of seven years, Biddy received her Free Certificate in July 1858. But she continued to struggle with colonial life. In February 1862 she was sent to prison for two months with hard labour for being idle and disorderly.

Biddy had brought her young daughter, Ann Daley, with her on the *Phoebe*. Ann was admitted to the Queen's Orphan School in 1846, when she was two. She had been there nearly thirteen years when she was apprenticed to Lawrence Cotham. She may have died as Ann McKenna, an Irish-born servant, who died in the

General Hospital, Hobart, in August 1868 of *mesenteric disease* (caused by drinking milk from cows infected with tuberculosis, causing tuberculosis of the lymph glands inside the abdomen—now rare as milk is pasteurised).

On 12 October 1863, after almost nineteen years in the colony, Biddy McKenna, a servant aged 54, died in the General Hospital, Hobart, of *carcinoma uteri* (cancer of the uterus).

SARAH
BROMLEY

Arriving in Van Diemen's Land in January 1829, Sarah Bromley's skills as a tailoress, dressmaker and cook were recorded, as well as her ability to make pastry. Such skills would have been in demand in the colony, just as they were in London. However, her husband had died leaving her to support two children. It may have been a struggle and on 10 April 1828 Sarah was indicted for having stolen two blankets value 9 shillings, two sheets value 2 shillings, one pillow value 4 shillings, one quilt value 2 shillings, one tablecloth value 1 shilling, and one candlestick value 6 pence of the goods of George Benjamin Poole of Charlotte Street, Somers Town in London. In an area of London once frequented by the likes of Charles Dickens and Mary

Shelley, Sarah rented a furnished back room belonging to George Poole. On 22 March she had dined with George's wife Mary, and afterwards was accused of taking the tablecloth. Three days later Mary suspected other items were missing and went to Sarah's room with a constable to demonstrate that a pair of sheets had also disappeared. Evidence was given by William Crush, a shopkeeper to a pawnbroker in Clarendon Square. He stated that Sarah had pawned two sheets on the 15th of the month, and the tablecloth on the day she dined with Mary. The other items she was accused of having stolen must have also come to light during the trial, as she was ultimately sentenced to transportation for seven years.

The *Harmony* took 123 days to travel to Hobart, arriving on 14 January 1829 with 100 female convicts on board plus 63 passengers, including 8 women and 33 children leaving their homeland to join their husbands. Sarah, travelling with her 12-year-old daughter Mary, was sufficiently educated to be appointed schoolmistress for children on the ship. Mary could read and write and her health on board was recorded as 'good'. On arrival, the widow Sarah at age 36 was described as having flaxen hair and eyebrows, a large oval head, perpendicular forehead, a large aquiline nose and she had lost two front teeth of her upper jaw.

It is not known whether Sarah's daughter Mary stayed with her as no reference is made to the child being accommodated at the Queen's Orphan School. Shortly after arrival Sarah found herself assigned in Hobart to the service of Dr William Bohan, military surgeon to the 63rd Regiment, and his wife. It might appear from Sarah's subsequent record of conduct that she could be mistaken for being of an insubordinate nature. The first offence of being insolent to her mistress was followed a few weeks later by gross misconduct—both offences bringing a sentence of confinement to a cell at the Cascades Female Factory on bread and water.

However, on returning to her service a month later on 19 November 1829, Sarah entered the Principal Superintendent's Office in Hobart with the intention of making a complaint against Dr and Mrs Bohan for ill-using her. She stated she had come to the office the day before for the same purpose, and did not return to the Bohan residence that evening but remained absent all night. She was ordered to the House of Correction and Second Class status until the case could be investigated. If an investigation took place it appears not to have gone in Sarah's favour as she was

returned to Dr Bohan's service.

At this time Dr Bohan worked as a medical attendant in Hobart, and also appeared as a juror on more than one occasion. In April 1830 Sarah absconded from his service, was apprehended, returned to the Female Factory for seven days in the cells on bread and water, then returned to the Bohan household. Contrary to other convicts who, after repeated misconduct in their assigned service, might be relocated to another master, Sarah was repeatedly returned to Dr Bohan. Four days after returning, she was brought before the magistrate again: 'insolence to her master and mistress and her absconding having caused her master considerable loss of property—cell on bread and water 6 days'. The offences that followed demonstrated a regular pattern of non-compliance, all while in the service of Dr Bohan. She neglected her work, left the house without leave, was disobedient and insolent. In 1831 a fellow servant John Spring who arrived on the *Marmion* in 1828 was tried at the Quarter Sessions on Saturday 18 June for having committed two offences, one of which was to steal two glass bottles and two half-pints of brandy of Dr Bohan's property. Found guilty, he was sentenced to 14 years. John was later removed to Port Arthur for another robbery and died there in September 1837.

A month after John's conviction for stealing brandy, Sarah committed her last offence in Bohan's service. Did she hope to break away once and for all? Creating a riot in the house appears to have done the trick as she was found neglectful of her duty and using improper language. The magistrate, stating that Sarah was clearly incorrigible, removed her to the Female Factory in July 1831 where she was placed in the Crime Class. She probably never saw Dr William Bohan again. In early 1832, his health appearing to wane, he was planning to proceed to Sydney, as an auction of his household furniture was advertised. However, he was still in Hobart in May when the *Hobart Town Courier* announced that as an 'eminent free-mason' he was appointed to the 'high station of Provincial Grand Master in Van Diemen's Land'. He was also known to associate with Port Arthur's Commandant Charles O'Hara Booth, Booth recording that he spent an evening with the Bohans on 13 May 1833. Dr Bohan's health may have improved and he departed for India with his regiment in 1834, but he died back in England at his residence in Regents Park on 9 September 1835.

Meanwhile, Sarah gained a Ticket of Leave in August 1832, and her Certificate of Freedom in March 1835. For whatever reason, she threatened her free status by stealing a cotton sheet the property of George Lowes in July 1840, for which she was sentenced to three months hard labour and placed in a separate working cell with the stipulation that it was not on bread and water. This was her last offence.

The last we know of Sarah is of her wedding day. On 1 March 1843 Sarah, now 47 years of age, joined with George Collins, 43 years old, a widower and blacksmith at St David's Church in Hobart before the Reverend William Bedford and two witnesses. Their fate is unknown.

♠9 ELIZABETH MAY

Elizabeth or Eliza May who arrived in Van Diemen's Land aboard the *Fame* was transported three times at least. So was Anna Scott who arrived on the *Borneo*. Elizabeth appears to be one of the women trapped in the revolving door of convict convictions. She stayed in the system for at least 40 years.

Elizabeth was first transported for Life to New South Wales in 1802, arriving on the *Atlas* as Eliza Dowling. She was from Kildare in Ireland and had been tried at the Kildare Summer

Sessions in 1801. She was a tall girl at 5 feet 5 inches with a ruddy, freckled complexion and dark brown hair and eyes. Her occupation was recorded as a country servant.

In 1805 Elizabeth married Laurence May, an Irish convict who arrived on the *Queen* in 1791. He was a successful farmer by 1804 when his first wife died from excessive drinking, leaving him in need of a nurse for his small children. Elizabeth and Laurence had two sons of their own. One son, Christopher, died in 1808 when he fell into a rain-filled sawpit when he was only four years old. Christopher Watkins May, born in 1813, made history in 1836 when he rode a velocipede down George Street in Sydney. In 1810 Elizabeth petitioned the Governor and as she was 'nine years an honest sober and unblemished character being lawfully married to Laurence May settler at the Hawkesbury', Governor Macquarie granted her freedom that was approved in 1815.

However something went wrong! Elizabeth and Laurence May separated by 1817 and Elizabeth arrived at Port Dalrymple in Van Diemen's Land aboard the *Fame*. Several offences were committed by Elizabeth in the colony during the 1820s. She was reprimanded, fined, sent to gaol and instructed to find sureties to keep the peace.

In New South Wales, Laurence was already living with Rosetta Kite and in 1817 their first son was born.

For some time, Elizabeth lived at Paterson's Plains with a man named Spencer. She said she was a widow when she was convicted in 1828, but in fact her husband was still alive in New South Wales. Why she came to Van Diemen's Land is not clear. Certainly, in the early days of settlement, there was movement between the colonies. Women were often landed at Sydney and then relocated to Van Diemen's Land. Sometimes records remain to give us a clear picture of what occurred, but not in Elizabeth's case. But we do know she was in the Port Dalrymple district and she was in trouble with the law, again. Tried at the Launceston Supreme Court in December 1828 with receiving stolen flour, she was prosecuted by Scott, the overseer for Mr J. Smith.

Her record is clear until 1831 when, being unfit for work, Elizabeth was returned to the House of Correction. She was reassigned and her next offence was for appearing drunk at the police office, not a very clever move. She spent four days in solitary with time to reflect on her behaviour. Alcohol played a part in her next sentence to transportation—in January 1832 she stole a quart of wine from her master, Mr Murray. She was tried at the Quarter Sessions and sentenced to seven years, her third sentence to transportation. In 1833 she was found to be drunk, useless and unable to do the work required of her resulting in time in the solitary working cells, and time at the wash tub. Elizabeth was returned to the Crown, not proving to be a reliable employee.

This pattern of behaviour continued throughout the 1830s. She spent another month in the solitary cells. Her last recorded offence was a charge of going about gossiping and begging. She had moved about the colony and was last recorded in the Richmond district. Elizabeth was a woman of perhaps 60 years of age. She had no family in Van Diemen's Land, no future. She was a product of a system that failed her. After her Certificate of Freedom was issued in 1840 nothing more was heard of her.

MARGARET
HAINES

According to Henry John Webb, giving evidence at the Proceedings of the Old Bailey on 17 September 1849, Margaret Haines stole money from him by putting her hand into his trouser pocket. They had been drinking and ate together earlier in the evening and he went 'home' with her to what was described as a brothel by the Police Sergeant giving evidence. Webb stated 'my trousers were on, I then felt in my pocket, and my money was gone'. Margaret denied the charge and though some money was in her possession the evidence was his word against hers. Her guilt appears to have been established by the Police Inspector who produced a certificate of a former conviction where she had served nine months for stealing a sovereign, and she was sentenced to transportation for seven years. Whether Margaret was a confirmed prostitute is unclear but this class of women has been described as 'artful and adroit thieves ... [where] they rifle his person when in the bedroom with him in low coffee-houses and brothels'. She was 47 years of age at the time, a literate housemaid and widow with four children. Her native place is listed as Paris where she may have lived previously, and at the time had a brother, and two sisters living in Cork, Ireland.

Margaret's circumstances may well have influenced her behaviour, having to find money to support herself and her children. But the fate of her children is unknown as there is no evidence they were with her when she arrived in Van Diemen's Land on the convict transport *St Vincent* (1) on 4 April 1850. Described as 'bad' on board, her continued rebelliousness led to repeated instances of incarceration for the next thirteen years.

As with most convict women, Margaret was assigned to a free settler on arrival. She worked for a variety of masters on the main streets of Hobart for an average of two to six weeks. Between stints of good behaviour Margaret committed a number of offences—insolence, drunkenness, being out after hours and disturbing the peace—and she was returned to the Female Factory in Hobart where she served periods of punishment ranging from two weeks to three months hard labour.

Her confinement at the womens' prison was marked by breaches of regulations including talking at muster, having items in her possession and loud talking. The Factory register of offences and punishments ordered also showed that on 16 September 1852 Margaret was charged for 'disorderly conduct at muster' and again for 'disorderly conduct' for which she was sentenced to 48 hours in the black hole for each offence. Reference to the 'black hole' is only found against Margaret's record in the register—it appears nowhere else. Reported in the British Parliamentary Papers on the subject of convict discipline and transportation, Superintendent of the Cascades Female Factory, J.M. May, wrote in his report dated 10 July 1852:

In order the more effectually to deal with prisoners [who offend], and to separate them entirely from every other prisoner in the establishment, and cut off every hope of communication, a "dumb cell" in a secluded part of the building has been authorized.

A 'dumb cell' or dark cell could well have been colloquially named 'black hole'. Since May's report was written just prior to Margaret's punishment it could well suggest that this cell was constructed, not just authorised, though it begs the question why it was not mentioned as a punishment for any other woman.

Margaret returned to assigned service and gained a Ticket of Leave in June of 1853 only to return to the Factory in late September of that year for common assault, for which she was sentenced to three months hard labour. Her Ticket was revoked and she was ordered not to enter service in Hobart. Back in confinement, her apartment was found to be dirty on two occasions and she was not performing her work—three days on bread and water was her punishment.

Her Ticket was returned in August 1854, only to be revoked again in November of that year for 'Having a man in her bedroom for an improper purpose'. For this she was sentenced to nine months hard labour and returned to the Female Factory. Margaret was recommended for a Conditional Pardon but she continued to reoffend. Nevertheless on 3 November 1856 she gained her Certificate of Freedom, just over seven years from the date of her original trial.

Free of the restrictions of convict life, her prospects were probably not that different 'on the outside', as most women exchanged life as a 'government' servant for one as a free servant. How she spent her life for the next two years is unknown but she appears to have married a man by the name of Coleman, and they lived in Campbell Street, Hobart. She charged a man for breaking windows of her residence in that street in March of 1858, but in November of that year, reference is made to a husband in court details following an offence she was convicted of, for which she received two years imprisonment with hard labour.

Tried as Margaret Coleman she was brought before the courts for assaulting Mrs Ann Wilks 'with intent to do her some grievous bodily harm by striking her on the head with a brass-headed whip' as *The Courier* described in October 1858. It appears that some ill-feeling existed between the two women. Mrs Wilks was walking home with her husband when they passed by Margaret's residence. *The Mercury* newspaper revealed that she came out and struck Ann rendering her insensible and proclaimed 'That settles you!'. The defence stated Mrs Wilks had brought it upon herself and though Margaret pleaded not guilty, the jury found to the contrary. However some members of the jury felt she should be granted mercy, but it was not to be. Returning to the Cascades Female Factory, she completed her sentence in September 1860. Her movements from then on are unknown, other than a reference on her conduct record showing that by 1863 she was at Port Sorell, east of Devonport where one final offence is recorded, 'Obtaining money by false pretences' for which she was sentenced to a further six months hard labour at the Launceston Female Factory. By then Margaret was 63 years of age.

MARY DEVEREUX

When the constables burst into the room, Mary Devereux was sitting on a flat fruit basket close to the fire and holding 'a lump of white stuff in her lap'. Nearby were the moulds she used to make counterfeit shillings.

'O Lord, it is all over with us now', she cried, and threw herself down on the floor. A policeman jumped on top of her and they struggled in the dark as Mary thrashed about, trying to pulverise a plaster-of-Paris mould by grinding it into pieces with her hip. The ruse didn't work, of course, and Mary Devereux was brought before the court at the Old Bailey, along with her 17-year-old daughter who had pleaded with the police when they were caught red-handed, 'Spare my mother, I don't care what becomes of me'. The court took a very dim view of counterfeiting the King's image on coins of the realm, and both mother and daughter were condemned to death, their sentences commuted to transportation for Life.

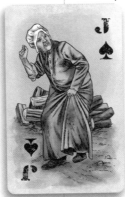

Mary Devereux the Elder—as she was designated in the convict records to distinguish her from her daughter Mary Devereux the Younger—was about 50 years old when she left England in June 1831 aboard a ship fittingly named the *Mary* (3). Her husband was dead, her son was transported for a separate offence, and her 10-year-old daughter Margaret was coming with her on the *Mary*, either willingly or unwillingly.

Upon arrival in Hobart Town, Mary the Elder was sent north, and her initial experiences of punishment were in the George Town Female Factory, which she visited three times in her first year. Three different employers brought her up on charges, first of disobeying her mistress's orders, then of being absent from her master's house without leave, and finally of 'grossly abusing her mistress & falsely accusing her of infidelity to her husband'. After this, Mary was sent south but the change in scenery made no difference to her behaviour, and from then on she was a frequent visitor to the Cascades Female Factory.

In many ways this 50-year-old convict behaved like a stereotype of the Irish woman she was, born around 1782 either in County Tipperary or County Tyrone (she gave different information on different occasions). She did not take kindly to authority and was charged again and again with being insolent, disobedient, or drunk. Between October 1831 when she arrived and January 1837, she had been sent to at least thirteen different households, and all had returned her to the Government on one of these charges. No one wanted her in the house, and given her record, that was understandable. But the Government didn't want to support her indefinitely either, and by 1838 she had been granted a Ticket of Leave.

The Government also did not want to support Mary's daughter Margaret any longer than necessary, and in November 1836 when Margaret was 15, she was discharged to her mother—who didn't have a Ticket of Leave at this time, and thus no way to earn money to support her daughter, even if she had been so inclined. Margaret, though totally innocent of any crime, upon arrival in Hobart had been sent to the Cascades Female Factory, where for more than a year she was confined to the Nursery Yard. Finally, on 9 January 1833, Margaret and another eighteen children were transferred from the convict nursery to the Orphan School in New Town. After being cooped up with infants (often sick or dying) and little children for so long Margaret may have found the Orphan School a relief. She may even have learned to read and write a little in the years she spent there. How she managed after she was discharged to her mother remains unknown.

Certainly her mother was not looking after her. Mary Devereux's stretches inside the Cascades Female Factory actually increased after she got her Ticket of Leave. In 1840 she was charged four times and had already spent seven months of the year inside before she was sentenced on 28 December to another six months hard labour. Whenever she was outside, she was probably destitute. Who would hire a woman like Mary? The older she grew, the less employable she was anyway. Mary was never a thief but she was a cranky old woman, and the Convict Department, to whom she was a nuisance, tried to keep her out of town. Because she had a Life sentence, she would have to be granted a Conditional Pardon to get out of the system, and her constant offending meant a series of Tickets of Leave granted, revoked, granted again, revoked again.

In February 1849, when Mary was in her late sixties, she was accused for the first time of actually inflicting damage on people and property. The charge was assault, and wilfully damaging windows to the amount of 10 shillings. She was 'fined 20/ for the assault and ordered to pay 10/ as compensation for injury done and costs, and in default of payment to be imprisoned 3 weeks'. Undoubtedly she defaulted and went to prison.

This would be the last time she was locked up. Later in the year she became quite ill, and was taken to the Colonial Hospital where she died on 25 November. She was buried as a pauper in the Catholic Burial Ground.

MARY
HICKEY

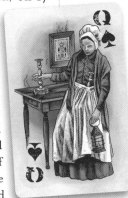

Mary Hickey was only 15 when she was tried on her first offence and sentenced to transportation for seven years for burglary. Having stolen candlesticks, she was tried in her home county, County Cork, on 17 February 1851. Very orderly and well-behaved during the voyage, she arrived at Hobart on the *John William Dare* on 22 May 1852.

Similar to many Irish convict women, Mary was single, Roman Catholic and illiterate. She also shared the common background of many Irish women who were transported, as Mary had no trade in Ireland but was allocated one when she arrived in Van Diemen's Land. Many younger girls, including Mary, were considered to be suitable for employment as nursemaids.

At just under five feet, Mary wasn't tall. She had a ruddy complexion, blue eyes, black hair and eyebrows, a small forehead and nose, and a large and thick mouth. She also had a mole on her right arm.

While under sentence, her conduct was almost blemish free. In October 1853 she was charged with disobedience of orders but the matter lapsed as no prosecutor appeared in the police court. In November 1854, she was granted a Ticket of Leave.

In February 1855 an application for marriage for Mary and Thomas Sblrwn [sic] was approved but does not appear to have taken place. She may have later married someone called Cooper but details of this are sketchy. In August 1855, Mary was recommended for a Conditional Pardon, and this was approved in July 1856.

Mary's later years in the colony were in stark contrast to her promising beginning. Perhaps she found life difficult once she was free. From 1856 to 1878, Mary did not appear in the colonial records. This changed in January 1878 when, as Mary Ann Cooper, she was fined 10 shillings 6 pence (or a fortnights imprisonment) for using obscene language. In February 1878 Mary appeared in the Hobart Police Office charged with larceny. She was sentenced to three months in the Female House of Correction. No sooner had she served her sentence when she was back in the Police Office in June 1878, this time charged with vagrancy. She had been found begging alms in the public street and received another sentence of three months in the Female House of Correction. This was to become the pattern of her life in her final years—prison, release, back to prison. In October 1878 she was again charged with larceny—stealing a pair of trousers from a shop—and was sent to prison for six months. She was then fined with three others for disturbing the peace in April 1879. The following month, as Mary Ann Hickey alias Cooper, she pleaded guilty in the Hobart Police Court to stealing a roll of tweed from a draper in Liverpool Street. She had cut the roll in two and attempted to pawn one half. Only recently released from gaol, she stated in her defence that she had not been right in her head since her husband died. Described as a confirmed thief, she was sent back to gaol for nine months. Was gaol her way of surviving? Her final sentence, of three months, was in May 1880 when she was charged with being idle and disorderly.

Described as 'an old woman', Mary Ann Cooper alias 'Hickle' died in tragic circumstances in December 1880, when she had only been out of gaol for a few days. The days leading up to her death were recorded in evidence given at her inquest. On Saturday night, she had paid for accommodation at Hopwood's lodging house in Lower Macquarie Street. Hopwood said she was drunk and that he knew her to be a woman

of drunken habits. A constable stated that he had heard sounds 'like faint woman's screams' that night and he searched the wharf but could not find anyone. Mary was found the following morning in the water near the Monarch Wharf. Her body was dragged out of the water and she was taken to the dead-house. The verdict of the inquest was that she was 'found drowned' but there was not sufficient evidence to show how she came into the water. She was only 44.

ANNE LOVELL

The pregnant Rachael Anne Ousten from Yorkshire had married Esh Lovell just two years before they sailed for Van Diemen's Land on the brig *Avon* with their infant Samuel. Recorded in most of the archival documents without her Christian name, on the voyage to Van Diemen's Land Anne gave birth to another son William Esh Lovell in Mauritius. They arrived in Hobart Town in July 1823. Anne was a dressmaker and milliner, Esh, a Wesleyan missionary and upon their arrival in Hobart the couple opened a store in Melville Street opposite the then new Wesleyan Chapel.

Esh and Anne placed an advertisement in the *Hobart Town Gazette* on 2 August 1823 listing the many and varied items they had for sale. The Lovell's emporium had all of the things the fledgling colonists may have required, offering up the following items:

Cape Madeira wine, dried fruits, sugar, butter, walnuts, almonds, slops of all kinds, Irish linen, bed furniture, black lead pencils, pins, needles, threads, tapes, cotton boxes, stockings, gloves, men's shoes and boots, &c; ironmongery, patent locks, door bolts and barrels, sheep and horse shears, knives, pit and hand saw files, scythes, sickles, and nails of various kinds and sizes.

The advertisement suggested that Esh, 'having had an opportunity of laying in the above Goods in London, the Cape of Good Hope, and the Isle of France, he presumes he can offer them at the lowest possible prices'. Whether it was lack of stock due to a sell-out sale or a growing business that made the Lovell's change location is not known, however, just two months after opening, they relocated to the corner of Elizabeth and Brisbane streets. Perhaps the move was a result of Anne's growing role in the business. The *Hobart Town Gazette* on 4 October 1823 stated 'in addition to a general store, Mrs. L. will carry on Dress Making, in all its various branches, in which commands will be thankfully received and duly executed. Also, a great number of caps, frills,

bonnets, and childrens' dresses are already on hand.'

The growth of the business might in fact have been the success of Anne's dressmaking. Within one month after the move to their new location, Anne placed a WANTED advertisement in the paper to engage two apprentices 'respectable young females' to her Millinery and Dressmaking business.

By September 1827, Anne now had five children—four sons and a daughter, and both she and Esh were heavily involved in the Wesleyan Church. Perhaps it was a combination of their work ethic and faith that, in the eyes of John Lakeland, Superintendent of Convicts, made them the ideal couple to place in charge of the soon to be established Cascades Female Factory.

Following the death of Mr Joshua Eynon Drabble, (the first Superintendent of the Hobart Gaol and Female Factory in Macquarie Street) the Colonial Government sought replacements to manage the female convicts, who, due to standards in the old gaol, were about to be moved to the newly refurbished distillery site in South Hobart.

Lakeland, in his letter to Lieutenant-Governor Arthur, recommended the Lovells, suggesting that managing the female convicts would require 'all the energy and nerve that any individual may possess'. Arthur instructed the Colonial Secretary to offer them the positions of Superintendent and Matron for a joint salary of £150 per annum as well as a house, wood, water and rations for the whole family.

The offer also stated that 'The main exertion will rest with the 'Matron' of the Establishment ... He [Esh] will be expected to offer Mrs. Lovell every assistance in the regulation of the accounts and ... the religious and moral direction of the institution'.

Anne and her husband were appointed on 29 February 1828 and moved into their accommodation, first at the Hobart Factory, then onto the Cascades prior to the transfer of the women from the Hobart site in the last days of December 1828. Just three months after moving, with the responsibility of managing the Factory on her shoulders, a pregnant Anne lost her second born son, William Esh Lovell, aged just 5 years. Three months passed and Anne gave birth to a daughter, again taking her brood to five. Many would consider having five children aged under five a full time job, however to Anne that was only half her role. The other half was managing an adult convict population of 200 plus, all the while living above the gateway of the Establishment in a small four room 'apartment'.

Anne's list of duties, as outlined by Lieutenant-Governor Arthur was unwavering:

The matron shall superintend such part of the employment of the women as falls within the province of a female, and shall attend to such matters as could not be properly performed by the Superintendent, and shall generally assist him in the care and control of the establishment ...

give instructions to the task women about the employment of the females ...

inspect the females in their separate wards at the morning muster, and shall see that they are clean and properly dressed ...

visit the sleeping rooms daily, and see that they are kept perfectly clean and in order ...

visit constantly throughout the day, the hospital, nursery and kitchen yards, and to superintend and give directions in all that is going forward in either, most watchfully observing that in every thing extreme cleanliness, and order, and industry, and economy prevail.

Perhaps the pressure all became a little too much for Anne, as in less than four years from taking the positions of Superintendent and Matron, Esh and Anne Lovell resigned. This came after a committee of inquiry into the Factory found faults with the loose classification of women under punishment and, among other things, Anne's occasional employment of needleworkers to serve the needs of her own family. With the inquiry into the punishment of convicts being carried out without any opportunity for Esh and Anne to defend themselves Esh objected to the committee's procedure, and the Lovells subsequently resigned when the inquiry ended in December 1831.

Little is known about the couple in the following three years, with the exception of Anne giving birth to another son named William Esh Lovell in Hobart in 1833. This appears to be during Esh's management of Prospect Place Academy, a seminary for young gentlemen in Murray Street. The following year Anne died at the age of 44, leaving behind her six children, the eldest only 12.

MARGARET
DALZEIL

Free society was expected to maintain a respectable face to the world, despite the somewhat disreputable surroundings of a convict colony at the end of the earth. And in a time of large families, frequent illness and few labour-saving devices, one or two household servants were indispensable. But sometimes they were more trouble than they were worth.

The *Glasgow Herald* of Friday 4 October 1850 reports that in June of that year, Margaret Dalzell [sic] and two female accomplices were charged with feloniously attacking James Robertson, striking him repeatedly

in the face, knocking him down and robbing him of a tin case containing a seaman's discharge and register ticket. Tried at the Glasgow Court of Justiciary on 30 September, all three women were sentenced to ten years transportation. Margaret had two prior convictions, one for stealing a watch, the other for housebreaking. Described as a Protestant housemaid from Glasgow who could read, she left behind two brothers and two sisters and arrived in Hobart in mid-1851 with her fellow partners in crime, on the *Aurora* (2) at the age of 20. At only 5 feet tall, with a ruddy complexion, brown hair, blue eyes and several tattoos, her general conduct on board was assessed as 'bad'.

First assigned to James Hurst, a former overseer of the Coal Mines on the Tasman Peninsula, she committed no offences in his household, but her next master was not so fortunate. From him she absconded and was sentenced to eight months hard labour at the Cascades Female Factory. In September 1852 she was assigned to James Calder—he was a man of many talents, surveyor, writer and artist, historian and ethnographer, but he could not manage Margaret. Within three days she had been charged with being drunk and out after hours and sentenced to six months hard labour at the Factory. For the next nine months she was in and out of the institution, and her record was marked 'not to be assigned south of Bridgewater'. Behind the Factory walls, repeated misdemeanours including insolence, neglect of duty and spilling oil in the ward led to sentences of bread and water and separate treatment.

By March 1853 Margaret was back in assigned service, and in April she applied for permission to marry convict William Hands, a whitesmith from Birmingham, but no recommendation from the clergy was forthcoming. In June of the same year she was sent to Daniel Stanfield at Clarence Plains, today's Rokeby, and almost immediately was in serious trouble there, charged with 'injuring her master's clothes' and sentenced to three months hard labour and returned to the Factory.

Her experience at the Female Factory was not without incident either. During this time, the institution's punishment books recorded a number of offences including insolence, breach of regulations in scrubbing the floor of her apartment before the regulation hour, and not being alert as watchwoman. Punishments included three days on bread and water, and one instance of ten days in separate treatment.

She continued to abscond from her next few places of assignment, receiving several more long sentences of hard labour until she relocated to Port Arthur in September 1856 and was assigned to the household of Mr Adolarius Boyd, Accountant and future Commandant. Female convicts did go to Port Arthur, but as assigned servants. At this relatively distant penal settlement, she was there less than two weeks before absconding while on pass from her service and was caught a week later. Where had she hidden, how had she fed herself and kept warm? Did she have help? We don't have the answers, but for her crime she was sentenced to a further 18 months of hard labour and returned to the Female Factory in Hobart.

After 14 months including further offences escalating from general misconduct, through refusing to attend prayers and assault—she appeared in December 1857 at the old Impression Bay Probation Station, where the typhus fever-stricken Scottish immigrants from the *Persian* emigrant ship were quarantined. She was presumably at work nursing them. Most of the victims were Highlanders who spoke only Gaelic and perhaps Margaret was one of the few available who could make herself understood to them and so was selected for this potentially fatal job? After about five weeks and ten deaths the Colonial Secretary was informed on 2 February 1858 that the station was closed, and Margaret received her Ticket of Leave on the very same day, a fitting reward for her courageous service.

In April 1858 she married former convict Robert Carter and they had three children—Robert, Mary Ann and James. According to her conduct record she remained on good behaviour for the next 16 years, apart from the occasional reference to being 'idle and disorderly'. However the newspapers provide two additional misdemeanours. In June 1871 it was alleged she burned the architraves of a house that was let to her husband Robert, who at the time was incarcerated in the Launceston House of Correction under a six month sentence. Though committed for trial, no further details are forthcoming.

Then in April of the following year, again before Magistrate Thomas Mason, she was charged with having her two sons Robert and James 'without means of support from the 24th July 1871'. She was remanded for a week, after which time it was determined that her husband had in fact had charge of them, and she was discharged. Subsequently, she was tried twice over the next few years under different names and at different places around the state—perhaps her marriage to Carter was over? And what of their daughter Mary Ann? We know that Robert died of a cancerous tumour in Launceston in June 1885.

It seems that Margaret had never managed to make a secure and comfortable life for herself. Her last court appearance for being idle and disorderly was in October 1882. Aged 52 it was now more than thirty years after she first set foot in Van Diemen's Land. Margaret had served a total of more than four years hard labour, including one sentence of eight months of which she was to spend each alternate month working in a separate cell. Her fate is unknown.

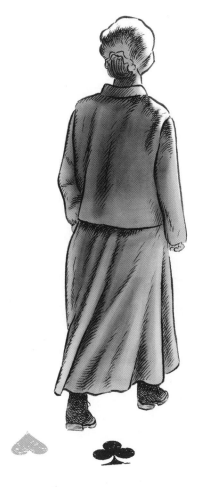

GLOSSARY

A

Anson: The HMS *Anson* arrived at Hobart as a male convict transport in 1844 and was subsequently refitted as a probation station for female convicts. It was then towed to Prince of Wales Bay, Risdon, near Hobart, where it was moored. This hulk housed female convicts during their six months probation upon arrival in Van Diemen's Land from 1844 to 1850.

Appropriation List: This convict record names the place or person to which the convict was first appropriated or assigned on arrival in Van Diemen's Land during the Assignment period.

Arthur, George: Lieutenant-Governor of Van Diemen's Land from 1824 to 1836. He continued the restructuring of the convict system started by his predecessor Colonel Sorell, a work that culminated in the founding of the Port Arthur penal station in September 1830. Recalled in 1836, he filled the appointment of Lieutenant-Governor of Upper Canada, and then Governor of the Presidency of Bombay in 1842 until forced to resign due to ill health in 1846. He died in September 1854.

Assignable Class: In the female factories, there were three classes of convicts. The assignable class (or first class) were those convicts who were able to be assigned (during the Assignment period) or hired as probation pass holders (during the Probation period). These were the best behaved convicts or those who had been returned by their employers for re-assignment.

Assignment System: The assignment system operated for female convicts from 1803 until 1843. Under this system, eligible convicts were assigned to employers (masters/mistresses) to work as domestic servants in return for accommodation, food and clothing. The convicts were not paid a wage and could be returned for re-assignment by their employer if they were no longer needed or were unsuitable.

B

Branch Factory: An off-site campus of a female factory; for example, Brickfields Hiring Depot.

Brickfields Hiring Depot: This hiring depot was situated at the Brickfields, New Town where North Hobart Oval and Rydges Hotel now stand. Female convicts eligible for assignment or hiring as probation pass holders were housed here between 1842 and 1852. It was a branch factory of Cascades Female Factory.

Brickfields Invalid Depot: See Brickfields Pauper Establishment.

Brickfields Pauper Establishment: Also known as Brickfields Invalid Depot, this was the same site as Brickfields Hiring Depot. It operated as an invalid depot for men from 1859 until 1882. The majority of inmates were ex-convicts.

C

Campbell Street Gaol: This gaol began in 1821 as convicts' barracks and from 1846 also served as a civilian prison. It became Hobart's main gaol in 1853 and the only gaol in the south from 1877 when Port Arthur closed. Campbell Street Gaol closed in 1960 when a new gaol was opened at Risdon.

Cascades Female Factory: This was the third-built female factory in Van Diemen's Land, after Hobart Town Female Factory and George Town Female Factory.

The first female convicts went to Cascades Female Factory in December 1828 and it operated as a female factory until 1856 when administration was passed to local authorities and it then operated as a gaol.

Cascades Gaol: Cascades Gaol was essentially the same establishment as Cascades Female Factory, but it operated under local authority administration from 1856 until its closure in 1877 when the remaining female prisoners were removed to Campbell Street Gaol.

Cascades Invalid Depot: The site of Cascades Female Factory operated as an invalid depot from 1867 until 1879, though women were only housed there until 1874 when they were removed to the New Town Pauper Establishment.

Central Criminal Court: Also known as the Old Bailey, this was the principle court for the City of London.

Certificate of Freedom: Convicts were eligible to receive a Certificate of Freedom (also known as a Free Certificate) when they had completed their sentence of transportation (but not if they were sentenced to Life). Not all convicts collected their Certificate of Freedom, and some only did so several years after their sentence expired. The Certificate allowed them to travel wherever they wished, restoring them to the privileges of the free.

Conditional Pardon: A convict became eligible to apply for a Conditional Pardon after a certain amount of their sentence had expired, or they had been sentenced to Life where a Certificate of Freedom would not be issued. Convicts applied at their local Police Office and it was granted by the Crown on the recommendation of the Lieutenant-Governor and approved if the convict was of good behaviour. A Conditional Pardon gave the

convict the status of a free person except that they were only allowed to travel within certain jurisdictions, usually the Australian colonies and New Zealand and were not permitted to return to the United Kingdom.

Conduct Record: This was the main convict record used by the Convict Department to record convict details including background history, marital status, transportation trial place, trial date, offence and sentence, colonial offences, locations and freedoms. Two different styles of conduct record exist, one for the convicts who arrived during the Assignment period, and a more detailed style for those who arrived during the Probation period. Probation period conduct records have the advantage of including religion, literacy, physical characteristics, age, trade and native place as well as more detailed information on the convict's locations during his/her time within the system. There is no difference between the appearance of the male and female conduct records, only the content. The original records are held at the Tasmanian Archive and Heritage Office (TAHO) as the CON 40 series for the assignment records and the CON 41 series for the probation records for female convicts.

Court of Justiciary: The name given to the Scottish court.

Crime Class: In the female factories this was the punishment class or third class. Convicts sentenced to the crime class undertook hard labour. After a certain portion of their sentence was served and they were of good behaviour, they could be moved to the second class. When their punishment sentence at the Female Factory was served they were moved to the assignable class for assignment or hiring.

D

Description List: This convict record was used by the Convict Department to record the physical characteristics of the convict, including any marks and their locations such as tattoos or freckles. The original records are held at the Tasmanian Archive and Heritage Office (TAHO) in the CON 19 series for female convicts and include details of height, hair and eye colour, size and shape of nose, mouth and chin, and may also include trade, age and native place.

Disorderly House: This usually referred to a brothel, but could also refer to an unlicensed grog shop. Often the two were combined.

Dissection: A practice undertaken in Van Diemen's Land on the bodies of murderers explicitly sentenced to be hanged and dissected, until 1869 when the *Act for Regulating the Practice of Anatomy* was passed. From 1869 the bodies of paupers or others who were unclaimed were also available for dissection for teaching and medical research.

Dynnyrne Nursery: This nursery operated from 1842 to 1851 at Dynnyrne House, South Hobart, not far from Cascades Female Factory. The establishment was run by Matron Slee.

Dysentery: An illness characterised by frequent, small-volume, severe diarrhoea which shows blood in the faeces along with internal cramping and painful straining to pass stools. Other symptoms include fever and malaise.

F

Female Factory: A house of correction for female convicts used as a place of punishment, confinement and hiring or assignment. While in the factory, convicts were expected to work at a range of tasks. There were five female factories in Van Diemen's Land: Hobart Town, George Town, Cascades, Launceston and Ross.

Female Orphan School: The female school at the Queen's Orphan School at New Town.

First Class: See Assignable Class.

Free Certificate: See Certificate of Freedom.

Free by Servitude: See Certificate of Freedom.

G

George Town Female Factory: This female factory operated on two sites in George Town in the early period of the colony from c.1822 to c.1834. It closed when the Launceston Female Factory opened.

H

Hard Labour: A punishment served in female factories, usually in the crime class. Two common forms of hard labour were washing clothes at the wash tub and picking oakum. The washing was often conducted in wet, cold conditions and was heavy work; picking oakum involved unravelling the hemp fibres from old tarry rope and often made the fingers bleed.

Hiring Depot: A place where employers could hire convicts into service. The main hiring depot for women was Brickfields in Hobart; though there were also hiring depots in Launceston and Ross. At one time, a hiring depot also operated from a house in Liverpool Street, Hobart.

Hobart Benevolent Society: Founded in 1832, the Hobart Benevolent Society aimed to help those in need, though it was always short of funds and its members preferred to help the deserving poor rather than malingers, drinkers or criminals. Due to lack of support it closed in 1839, but re-opened in 1860.

Hobart Gaol, Campbell Street: See Campbell Street Gaol.

Hobart Town Female Factory: This female factory opened in 1822 and operated until January 1829 when the last of the inmates were removed to Cascades Female Factory. It adjoined Old Hobart Gaol.

Hobart Town Gaol, Macquarie Street: See Old Hobart Gaol.

House of Correction: A place of punishment for convicts charged with offences (usually against convict discipline). Female factories were houses of correction.

Hulk: A hulk was a prison ship. Usually these ships were no longer sea worthy and were converted to house convicts in a floating prison. The *Anson* hulk was used as a probation station for female convicts near Hobart.

I

Indent: This convict record was one of the three main documents the colonial authorities used to record details of convicts. Indents were not as detailed as conduct records and repeated a lot of the same information. However, indents provided information on living relatives of the convicts such as the name of parents and siblings. Most of these records are held at the Tasmanian Archive and Heritage Office (TAHO) in the record series CON 15 for female convicts. Some of the indents are held in the Mitchell Library in Sydney.

Infant School: One of the schools which made up the Queen's Orphan Schools. It catered for children from about three to seven years of age.

Interior: Any part of Van Diemen's Land outside the two main centres, Hobart and Launceston. Convicts were often sent to the interior to remove them from bad influences in the towns.

Iron Collar: This was a punishment device. Made of heavy iron, it circled the neck and had spikes radiating from it. The spikes made it uncomfortable for the prisoner to lie down.

K

King's Orphan School: Established in 1828 and later to become the Queen's Orphan School in line with the reigning monarch of the time. See Queen's Orphan School.

L

Launceston Female Factory: This female factory opened in November 1834, replacing the George Town Female Factory. It closed in 1855, but then continued to operate as a women's prison. It was situated on the site of the present-day Launceston College, next to the men's gaol.

Launceston Gaol: This was the same establishment as the Launceston Female Factory after it ceased to operate as a female factory, with control handed over to the local authorities. There was also a Launceston Gaol for male prisoners, next door.

Light Working Cells: See Separate Working Cells.

M

Male Orphan School: This was the male school at the Queen's Orphan Schools.

Millbank Penitentiary: This was a large penitentiary situated on the Thames River, London which opened in 1821. It was demolished in 1890 and the Battersea Power Station built on the site, now the Tate Britain art gallery. Silent treatment was the main form of control used in the penitentiary, which had a male and a female section.

N

New Norfolk Insane Asylum: This hospital was built in 1829 located near Willow Court in the Royal Derwent Hospital precinct at New Norfolk. The site was used as a mental hospital from 1833 until 2000–2001.

New Town Charitable Institution: This was an invalid depot which mainly housed ex-convicts, and operated on the site of the Queen's Orphan Schools at New Town from 1874 for women and from 1879 for men.

New Town Farm: New Town Farm was attached to the Queen's Orphan Schools complex. It operated mainly as a farm for the Queen's Orphan Schools, but also at various times as a probation station and a nursery. Many boys were relocated here on their discharge from the Point Puer Boys' Establishment at Port Arthur.

New Town Invalid Depot: See New Town Charitable Institution.

New Town Pauper Establishment: See New Town Charitable Institution.

Nursery: Many female convicts brought young children with them when they were transported, or bore children (often illegitimate) while under sentence. Those under three years of age were usually housed in a nursery. At various times the nurseries were part of the female factories and at others were in separate institutions, especially in Hobart, where nurseries existed at various times in a house in Liverpool Street, at Dynnyrne House, at Brickfields and at New Town Farm.

O

Old Bailey: (see Central Criminal Court)

Old Hobart Gaol: This was the first gaol built in Hobart, in 1817, and was located on the south-west corner of Macquarie and Murray Streets. It mainly housed male prisoners, but before the Hobart Town Female Factory opened there was a room for female prisoners. The gallows were located in the yard of the gaol. The gaol closed in 1854.

On the Town: This phrase normally meant that the female convict had worked as a prostitute.

P

Permission to Marry: From 1829 to 1857, convicts in Van Diemen's Land were required to seek permission to marry from the Lieutenant-Governor, even if only one of them was a convict. It was usually the male who made the application.

Port Arthur: The Port Arthur penal settlement on the Tasman Peninsula operated from 1830 to 1877. It catered predominantly for re-offending male convicts, but not all were serious offenders, many sent there for absconding or refusing to work. In its latter years of operation, the aged and infirm were also sent there. Some female convicts were at Port Arthur as assigned servants to officials at the settlement.

Prison Hulk: See Hulk.

Probation: From 1844 until the end of transportation in 1853, female convicts were required to serve six months probation upon arrival in Van Diemen's Land. This probation period was designed to teach convicts desirable skills—including reading, writing, ciphering (numeracy), needlework, domestic service—and also to separate the newly arrived convicts from the more hardened criminals in the female factories. When the six months probation was completed, a convict became a probation pass-holder.

Probation Pass-holder: A probation pass-holder was able to be hired to work by an employer. A class-based indulgence reflecting good conduct, convicts were paid a minimum wage of £7 per annum.

Probation Station: A probation station was where convicts completing their six months probation period were housed and worked. For male convicts, probation stations were dotted all over Van Diemen's Land. For female convicts, the *Anson* hulk was the main probation station. New Town Farm operated temporarily as a probation station for female convicts in 1850.

Q

Queen's Orphan School(s): This institution comprised three schools—the male school, the female school and the infant school. It was located at New Town in what is now known as the St John's Park precinct. Children of convicts were sent there when they arrived on convict transports or when their mother was under punishment.

Queen's Orphanage: See Queen's Orphan School(s).

R

Ross Female Factory: This female factory opened in March 1848 and closed in November 1854.

Ross Hiring Depot: This hiring depot operated from within the Ross Female Factory.

S

Second Class: Prisoners in the second class at a female factory were those working their way up from third (or crime) class to first class, those imprisoned for minor offences (i.e. not undertaking hard labour) and those awaiting confinement.

Separate Apartments: These punishment cells were located in Yard 3 at Cascades Female Factory. They were completely dark when both the inner and outer doors were shut and locked. Silence prevailed in these apartments.

Separate Working Cells: These were solitary confinement cells which allowed light in above the door so that prisoners could work, probably at picking oakum (see Hard Labour for a description) or suchlike, while in confinement. They were situated in Yard 3 at Cascades Female Factory.

Solitary Cells: These were cells in female factories and gaols where prisoners would be kept apart from others. They were usually dark and cramped.

Solitary Confinement: This punishment kept a prisoner separate from all other prisoners, locked in a small dark cell or separate apartment. They were often fed only on bread and water while in solitary confinement. The maximum number of days a prisoner could spend in solitary confinement at one stretch was fourteen.

Solitary Working Cells: See Separate Working Cells.

Surgeon Superintendent: This was the medical attendant on board transport ships. He was responsible both for the medical care of the convicts and for their discipline.

Surgeon's Journal: This document was recorded by the Surgeon Superintendent on board the convict ship during the voyage. It included a sick list, records of cases in the hospital and general remarks. The journals are part of the Admiralty (ADM) series of British records and microfilmed as part of the Australian Joint Copying Project.

T

Third Class: See Crime Class.

Ticket of Leave: An indulgence given at the Lieutenant-Governor's discretion, it entitled the convict to work for wages and for whom they chose. Usually granted after the convict had served at least three years, it was the first step towards freedom, but it often restricted them to a particular police district and a requirement to attend a regular 'muster'. A little like parole today.

V

Visiting Magistrate: Several visiting magistrates operated across the colony. They visited hiring depots, gaols and female factories to pass sentence on prisoners charged with major crimes within the establishments.

W

Wash Tub: This was a punishment usually given when female convicts were sentenced to hard labour. Female convicts worked at the wash tub in Yard 2 at Cascades Female Factory washing clothes and linen. It was difficult, heavy, wet and cold work.

Working Yards: These were the yards at the female factories where prisoners worked, mainly at washing.

Sources

KEY

BDM	Birth, Death or Marriage registrations
BPP	British Parliamentary Papers
CCC	Proceedings of trials at the Central Criminal Court (Old Bailey), London—viewed via www.oldbaileyonline.org
LMA	London Metropolitan Archives
MF	Microfilm
NRS	National Records of Scotland
QVMAG	Queen Victoria Museum and Art Gallery, Launceston
SLNSW	Mitchell Library, State Library New South Wales
SRNSW	State Records New South Wales
TAHO	Tasmanian Archive and Heritage Office
TNA	The National Archives (UK)

CONVERSION TABLE

1 inch	2.5 centimetres
1 foot	0.3 metres
1 yard	0.9 metres
1 mile	1.6 kilometres
1 acre	0.4 hectare
12d (12 pence)	1 shilling
20s (20 shillings)	£1 (1 Pound)
1 gallon	4.5 litres
1 ounce	28 grams
1 pound	450 grams

HEARTS

2 Hearts - Mary Derrick
Newspapers: *Liverpool Mercury* (Liverpool, England) 6 Jun 1848; *Cornwall Chronicle* 24 Jun 1854, p. 8—TAHO: CON 41-1-27 no. 718; CON 15-1-6 pp. 178-179; CON 19-1-8; CON 33-1-97 no. 22825.

3 Hearts - Mary Ann Wood
TAHO: CON 41-1-6 no. 639; CON 15-1-3 pp. 176-177; CON 19-1-5; CON 33-1-39 no. 9404; CON 52-1-6.

4 Hearts - Bridget Hehir
BDM (TAHO): RGD 33-1-4 Birth Hobart 1383/1852; RGD 33-1-6 Birth Hobart 1978/1856; RGD 33-1-8 Birth Hobart 4455/1861; RGD 33-1-8 Birth Hobart 5703/1862; RGD 33-1-9 Birth Hobart 8493/1866; RGD 35-1-3 Death Hobart 1482/1852; RGD 35-1-5 Death Hobart 983/1858; RGD 35-1-7 Death Hobart 6174/1866; RGD 35-1-14 Death Hobart 1404/1894; RGD 37-1-15 Marriage Hobart 191/1856—Newspapers: *The Mercury* 9 May 1867 p. 2; 16 Oct 1868 p. 2; 15 Feb 1871 p. 2; 2 Mar 1871 p. 2; 5 Jul 1871 p. 2; 13 Jul 1871 p. 3; 1 Aug 1871 p. 2; 24 Aug 1871 p. 2; 3 Oct 1871 p. 2; 14 Nov 1871 p. 3—TAHO: CON 41-1-30 no. 885; CON 15-1-7 pp. 29-30; CON 19-1-9; ADM 101-12 Reel 3189; MM 71-1-1; CON 52-1-7 p. 3; CON 52-1-7 p. 258; CON 52-1-7 p. 362; CON 33-1-23 no. 5435.

5 Hearts - Mary Ann Haldane.
BDM (TAHO): RGD 36-1-2 Marriage New Norfolk 1711/1831; RGD 37-1-19 Marriage Hobart 184/1860; RGD 37-1-20 Marriage Hobart 155/1861; RGD 35-1-4 Death Hobart 1783/1855; RGD 35-1-5 Death Hobart 1126/1858; RGD 35-1-9 Death Hobart 1986/1879—Books: Rosner 2010—Newspapers: *Caledonian Mercury* 10 Nov 1827; *Colonial*

Times 17 Aug 1841, p. 2; *Tasmanian Police Gazette* 11 Nov 1881, p. 180—**NRS**: AD 14-27-17; AD 14-27-62 (courtesy A Davidson)—**TAHO**: CON 40-1-3 p. 33; CON 40-1-5 p. 61; CON 31-1-1 p. 54; CON 45-1-1 p. 5; SC 195-1-42-4338; SC 195-1-5-262—**Web**: http://malham-rennie.blogspot.com.au/2012/10/a-lucky-escape-mary-ann-haldane.html.

6 Hearts - Sarah Mason
BDM (TAHO): RGD 35-1-59 Death New Norfolk 989/1890—**Newspapers**: *Hobarton Mercury* 5 Jan 1857 p. 2—**Misc**: BPP 1869, p. 68—**TAHO**: CON 41-1-3 no. 1286; CON 15-1-7 pp. 107-108.

7 Hearts - Mary Devign
Books: Tardif 1990, p. 1260—**TAHO**: CON 40-1-3 p. 44; CON 31-1-10 p. 51; CON 19-1-13 p. 427.

8 Hearts - Sarah Jacobs
Books: Elias 2003; Frost 2012 pp. 76-77; Levi 2006 pp. 353-54; Phillips 1855; Tardif 1990 pp. 1283-1286—**CCC**: Trial of Sarah Jacobs (t18270913-158)—**Newspapers**: *Morning Chronicle* 17 Sep 1827; *Hobart Town Courier* 29 Oct 1831; *Colonial Times* 2 Nov 1831; 7 May 1839—**TAHO**: CON 40-1-5 p. 23; CON 32-1-2 p. 126; CON 32-1-5 p. 98; CON 19-1-13 p. 437; MM 33-1-1; MM 33-1-3; MM 33-1-5.

9 Hearts - Nappy Ribbon
BDM (TAHO): RGD 33-1-25 Birth Launceston 3011/1851; RGD 33-1-32 Birth Launceston 491/1854; RGD 35-1-23 Death Campbell Town 268/1854; RGD 37-1-17 Marriage Port Sorell 706/1858—**Books**: Bateson 1983 p. 393; Frost 2011 p. 18; Williams 1994 pp. 26, 66, 107, 122—**News-**

papers: *Hobarton Mercury* 2 Apr 1855 p. 2; *Launceston Examiner* 30 Jun 1870 p. 6—**TAHO**: CON 41-1-20 no. 475; CON 15-1-5 pp. 116-117; CON 33-1-88 no. 20276; CON 52-1-5 p. 60.

10 Hearts - Mary McLauchlan
Books: Goc 2013 pp. 97-124; MacDonald 2005 pp. 42-85—**Newspapers**: *Glasgow Herald* 25 Apr 1828; *Colonial Times* 16 Apr 1830, 23 Apr 1830; *Tasmanian and Austral-Asiatic Review* 16 Apr 1830, 23 Apr 1830; *Hobart Town Courier* 17 Apr 1830, 24 Apr 1830—**NRS**: Minutebook of Trial, High Court of Justiciary JC 26-1828-263; Precognition against Mary McLachlan [sic] for theft, AD 14-28-161; Precognition against Mary McLauchlane [sic] for theft, AD 14-28-203—**TAHO**: CON 40-1-5 p. 43; CON 19-1-13 p. 29; MM 33-1-1; MM 33-1-3; SC 41-1-1-143; Minutes of Proceedings of the Executive Council, Apr 1830, EC 4-1-1.

Jack of Hearts - Mary Wilkes
Books: Melville 1833—**TAHO**: CON 40-1-9 p. 283; CON 31-1-42 p. 90; CON 23-1-3; ADM 101-69 Reel 3210—**Web**: 'Anstey, Thomas (1777–1851)'. Australian Dictionary of Biography, National Centre of Biography, Australian National University, http://adb.anu.edu.au/biography/anstey-thomas-1709/text1859 [accessed 31 Aug 2013].

Queen Hearts - Mary Kennedy
BDM (TAHO): RGD 33-1-7 Birth Hobart 1481/1858; RGD 35-1-7 Death Hobart 4977/1865; RGD 37-1-15 Marriage Hobart 265/1856—**Books**: Abbott & Hall 1865 pp. 37-38; Chick 2009 p. 185; Grundy 2006 p. 62—**TAHO**: CON 41-1-31 no. 450; CON 15-1-7 pp. 101-102; CON 138-1-1

CLUBS

pp. 127-130; CON 138-2-1 pp. 93-94, 96-97; CON 52-1-6, CON 52-1-7 p. 158—**Web**: The Terry and Read family http://www.theforsterfamily.com/The%20Terry%20and%20Read%20Families.pdf [accessed 20 Feb 2014].

King of Hearts - Elizabeth Cato

BDM (LMA): Saint Mary at Lambeth, Register of Marriages, P85-MRY1, item 402—**Books**: Levy 1953; Rayner 1981—**Newspapers**: *Colonial Times* 1 Feb 1831 p. 2, 7 Sep 1832 pp. 3-4, 13 Mar 1838 p. 5&7, 20 Mar 1838 pp. 5-6, 3 Apr 1838 p. 6, 11 Apr 1843 p. 2; *Sydney Gazette & NSW Advertiser* 17 Apr 1841 p. 2—**Misc**: *The Athenaeum- Journal of literature, science, and the fine arts*, Jan to Dec 1831. J. Lection, London 1831; Genealogical Society of Tasmania Inc., Australia Cemetery Index, 1808-2007—**Web**: Weald of Kent, Surrey and Sussex Database ver. 10.03, http://www.theweald.org/home.asp [accessed 3 Jan 2014).

Ace of Hearts - Sarah Newall

Newspapers: *Cornwall Chronicle* 20 Mar 1861 p. 3, 30 Mar 1861 pp. 4-5, 10 Apr 1861 p. 5, 18 May 1861 p. 5, 2 Jul 1873 p. 3, 24 Jan 1876 p. 4; *Launceston Examiner* 2 Apr 1861 p. 4, 5 May 1868 p. 5, 14 Feb 1882 p. 3, 15 Feb 1882 p. 2, 16 Feb 1882 p. 2, 18 Feb 1882 p. 2—**TAHO**: CON 41-1-3 no. 216; CON 15-1-7 pp. 115-116; ADM 101-6 Reel 3189.

2 Clubs - Elizabeth Roberts

BDM (TAHO): RGD 33-1-2 Birth Hobart 1703/1846; RGD 33-1-3 Birth Hobart 1095/1848; RGD 33-1-4 Birth Hobart 203/1851; RGD 33-1-5 Birth Hobart 375/1853 —**Books**: Purtscher 1994—**Newspapers**: *Cornwall Chronicle* 23 Jan 1847, 14 Sep 1869; *Colonial Times* 2 Sep 1851, 1 Feb 1853, 28 Jun 1853, 29 Oct 1853, 11 Apr 1855; *Launceston Examiner* 18 Feb 1852, 28 Jun 1855; *Courier* 21 Apr 1852, 23 Jan 1855, 5 Feb 1855, 7 May 1858; *Hobarton Mercury* 9 Sep 1854, 11 Oct 1854, 24 Jan 1855, 12 Mar 1855, 9 May 1855, 10 Oct 1856, 10 Oct 1858; *Hobart Town Daily Mercury* 4 Feb 1857, 6 Oct 1859; *Mercury* 14 Jan 1862, 11 Jan 1864, 29 Oct 1864, 13 Oct 1865, 8 Feb 1868, 11 Aug 1868—**TAHO**: CON 40-1-8 p. 281; CON 19-1-2; CON 31-1-2 p. 74; CON 18-1-8 p. 288; CON 37-1-10 p. 5760; CON 52-1-2 p. 8; SWD 28; SC 195-1-41-4251.

3 Clubs - Ann Catchlove

BDM (TAHO): RGD 33-1-5 Birth Hobart 1434/1854; RGD 35-1-4 Death Hobart 1659/1855; RGD 37-1-13 Marriage New Norfolk 1208/1854—**SRNSW**: Inward passenger lists, series 13278, reels 399-560, 2001-2122, 2751—**TAHO**: CON 41-1-32 no. 1197; CON 15-1-7 pp. 147-148; CON 19-1-10; CON 138-1-1 p. 35; CON 33-1-105 no. 25072; HSD 246-1-9 vol. 13 folios 88, 140—**TNA**: HO 107, piece 1655, folio 201, p. 34 UK Census 1851 Westbourne, Sussex.

4 Clubs - Bridget Murphy

BDM (TAHO) RGD 35-1-61 Death Launceston 83/1892—**Newspapers**: *Launceston Examiner* 13 Jul 1871 p. 5, 18 Feb 1873 p. 2 supp, 9 Mar 1878 p. 3, 2 Jul 1879 p. 3, 4 Nov 1885 p. 3, 18 Mar 1892 p. 4, 18 Mar 1892 p. 4; *Mercury* 24 May 1886 p. 3—**TAHO**: CON 41-1-12 no. 737; CON 15-1-4 pp. 66-67.

5 Clubs - Sarah Baker
BDM (TAHO): RGD 33-1-30 Birth
Campbell Town 110/1852; RGD 33-1-44
Birth Deloraine 274/1866; RGD 35-1-2
Death Hobart 2328/1849; RGD 35-1-38
Death Westbury 543/1869—**Newspapers**:
Exeter & Plymouth Gazette 26 Mar 1842; *Western Times* 26 Mar 1842; *The Cornwall Royal Gazette, Falmouth Packet and Plymouth Journal* 25 Mar 1842, issue 3988; *Colonial Times* 29 Aug 1855; *Mercury* 2 Mar 1861 p. 2, 3 Nov 1868; *Cornwall Chronicle* 7 Jul 1866—**Misc**: QVMAG Baptismal Records; Cornwall Family History Society, database, baptisms—**TAHO**: CON 40-1-2 p. [112]; CON 15-1-2 pp. 4-5; CON 19-1-3; ADM 101-65 Reel 3209; GO 33-44 p.1; CON 44-1-5 Sep 1833, Oct 1864 (1848); SWD 26-1-4; SWD 27-1-1; SWD 32-1-1.

6 Clubs - Isabella Munro
Newspapers: *Cornwall Chronicle* 15 Feb 1860 p. 5, 20 Aug 1862 p. 6, 13 Sep 1862 p. 5, 13 Jun 1863 pp. 2-3, 3 Oct 1863 p. 3, 10 Oct 1863 p. 9, 21 Oct 1863 p. 3, 28 Oct 1863 p. 5, 2 Jan 1864 p. 3, 25 Oct 1865 p. 4, 30 Aug 1865 p. 5, 24 Feb 1866, p. 3, 19 May 1866 p. 4, 2 Mar 1867 p. 5, 13 Mar 1867 p. 4, 20 Mar 1867 p. 5, 30 Oct 1867 p. 5, 13 May 1868 pp. 4-5, 27 Apr 1870 p. 3; *Launceston Examiner* 14 Aug 1862 p. 5, 21 Aug 1862 p. 3, 25 Sep 1862 p. 3, 27 Sep 1862 pp. 2-3, 16 May 1863 p. 2, 28 May 1863 p. 2, 11 Jun 1863 p. 3, 1 Oct 1863 p. 3, 10 Oct 1863 pp. 2-3, 28 Oct 1863 p. 5, 29 Oct 1863 p. 3, 5 Jan 1864 p. 3, 28 Mar 1865 p. 5, 2 Nov 1865 p. 3, 30 Dec 1865 p. 4, 16 May 1866 p. 3, 14 Mar 1867 p. 5, 18 May 1867 p. 5, 30 Oct 1867 p. 5, 12 May 1868 p. 3; *Mercury* 17 Oct 1865 p. 1—**NRS**: Trial transcript JC26-1840-324—**TAHO**: CON 41-1-31 no. 1298; CON 15-1-7 pp. 111-112.

7 Clubs - Lydia Gordon
BDM (TAHO): RGD 37-1-12 Marriage
Hobart 591/1853—**CCC**: Trial of Lydia

Gordon (t18501021-1754)—**Newspapers**:
Launceston Examiner 17 Jan 1857 p. 3—**TAHO**:
CON 41-1-31 no. 559; CON 15-1-7 pp.
91-92.

8 Clubs - Mary Leary
BDM (TAHO): RGD 35-1-8 Death Hobart
992/1872; RGD 35-1-8 Death Hobart
2263/1874; RGD 37-1-2 Marriage Brighton
1424/1842; RGD 37-1-15 Marriage Richmond 852/1856—**Misc**: National Archives of
Ireland TR3 p. 305—**TAHO**: CON 40-1-6
p. [298]; CON 19-1-1; CON 52-1-2 p.
131; CON 52-1-6 18 May 1853, CON 52-1-7 p. 532.

9 Clubs - Rebecca Daynes
BDM (TAHO): RGD 33-1-3 Birth Hobart
2392/1850; RGD 35-1-3 Death Hobart
135/1850; RGD 37-1-10 Marriage Spring
Bay 936/1851—**Newspapers**: *Brisbane Courier* 15
Nov 1893 p. 2—**TAHO**: CON 41-1-13 no.
566; CON 15-1-4 pp. 90-91; CON 52-1-3
p.22; CON 52-1-3 p. 300; CON 52-1-4;
SC 195-1-30-2699 p. 10—**TNA**: Class:
HO 27, piece: 6, p.287 Norfolk Criminal
Register 1845—**Web**: 'Edward Deans', www.
orphanschool.org.au [accessed 21 Dec
2013].

10 Clubs - Mary Shaw
BDM (TAHO): RGD 35-1-37 Death
Kingston 258/1868—**Books**: Coxe 1825;
Tardif 1990, pp. 1697-1698—**TAHO**: CON
40-1-9 p. [72]; CON 19-1-1 p. 402.

Jack of Clubs - Catherine Owens
Books: Frost 2001 pp. 79-90; Frost 2012—
Newspapers: *Lancaster Gazette* 7 Mar 1829, 21
Mar 1829; *Cornwall Chronicle* 22 Oct 1842—
TAHO: CON 40-1-7 p. [4]; CON 32-1-1
p. 115; CON 32-1-4 p. 33; CON 19-1-13;
MM 33-1-1; MM 33-1-3; MM 33-1-5; MM
33-1-7; MM 33-1-8; CSO 22-1-50; LC
83-1-2.

Queen of Clubs - Elizabeth Payne
Book: Tardif 1990, pp. 1096, 1757—**News**

papers: *Hobart Town Courier* 19 May 1832, 18 Oct 1833—**TAHO**: CON 40-1-7 p. 24; SC 195-1-37-3671.

King of Clubs - Mary Hutchinson
Books: Daniels 1998; Frost 2013 pp. 38-67; Gunson 1967 pp. 290-91; Hutchinson 1961 pp. 93-108; Hutchinson 1965 pp. 50-67; Stringer 1885; Wright & Clancy 1993—**Newspapers:** *Colonial Times* 13 Mar 1838, 20 Mar 1838, 27 Mar 1838, 3 Apr 1838; *Hobart Town Gazette* 3 Oct 1829—**SLNSW:** Schofield, William. Letterbook 31 Dec 1827-5 Nov 1839, MF: ML B862; Thomas, John. "Official Journal of Rev. John Thomas", ML MSS 6228 item 1; Thomas, John. "Private Journal of Rev. John Thomas", ML MSS 6228 item 2; Thomas, John. "A Memoir of Sarah Thomas", ML MSS 6228 item 3; Thomas, Sarah. "Private Journal of Sarah Thomas", ML MSS 6228 item 4; Turner, J. G. "Diary of J G Turner", MF: reel CY 120—**TAHO:** Denison to Lord Grey 3 Jul 1851 GO 33 pp. 705-12; CSO 1-902-19161.

Ace of Clubs - Margaret Shaw
Books: Cowley & Snowden 2013—**CCC:** Trial of Margaret Shaw (t18400914-2357)—**Newspapers:** *Hobart Town Gazette* 13 Oct 1843 p.1122—**SLNSW:** MF: CY 1282; MF: CY 1197 p.151; MF: CY 958 p. 440—**TAHO:** CON 40-1-10 p. 49; CON 19-1-1; SC 195-1-11-916; CSO 22-1-112 folio 2385 no.1829-1, 25 Jul 1844; CSO 22-1-112 folio 2385 no.2273-3, 31 Oct 1844; ADM 101-63 Reel 3208.

2 Diamonds - Elizabeth Ferguson
BDM (TAHO): RGD 37-1-7 Marriage Hobart 1707/1848—**Newspapers:** *The Argus* (Melbourne) 17 Sep 1862 p. 7; 19 Sep 1862 p. 6; 24 Aug 1869 p. 6—**TAHO:** CON 41-1-4 no. 298; CON 15-1-3 pp. 60-61.

3 Diamonds - Melorina Florentina de Saumarez
Newspapers: *Morning Post* 14 Nov 1846; *Northern Star* 14 Nov 1846; *Hampshire Telegraph* 9 Jan 1847; *Cornwall Chronicle* 10 Jan 1876—**TAHO:** CON 41-1-13 no. 565.

4 Diamonds - Honorah Sullivan
BDM (TAHO): RGD 37-1-13 Marriage Hobart 655/1854—**Books:** Snowden, 2005—**Newspapers:** *Mercury* 7 Jun 1913 p. 5—**TAHO:** CON 41-1-35 no. 1057; CON 15-1-7 pp. 349-350; CON 52-1-6; CON 52-1-7 p. 404; CON 33-1-101 no. 24020; CON 14-1-42 pp. 212-213.

5 Diamonds - Mary Murphy
TAHO: CON 41-1-22 no. 996; CON 15-1-5 pp. 222-223; CON 19-1-7.

6 Diamonds - Grace Heinbury
Books: Frost 2001 pp. 79-90, Frost 2012—**Newspapers:** *Leicester Journal, and Midland Counties General Advertiser* 26 Jun 1837, 30 Jun 1837, 4 Aug 1837; *Hobart Town Gazette* 29 Jun 1838, 14 Dec 1838, 19 Apr 1839, 11 Oct 1839, 3 Jan 1840, 7 Aug 1840, 12 Mar 1841, 9 Apr 1841, 15 Oct 1841, 25 Feb 1842; *Hobart Town Courier and Van Diemen's Land Gazette* 11 Oct 1839; *Launceston Examiner* 16 Apr 1842—**TAHO:** CON 40-1-6 p. [16]; MM 33-1-4; MM 33-1-6; MM 33-1-8; Report of the Committee of Inquiry into Female Convict Prison Discipline CSO 22-1-50; ADM 101-16 Reel 3189; Tasmania Pardons 1841-1842 AJCP HO 10/51.

7 Diamonds - Eliza Benwell
Books: MacDonald 2006—**CCC:** Trial of Eliza Benwell (t18350511-1275 and

t18350511-1276)—**Newspapers:** *Colonial Times* 23 Apr 1830, 12 Sep 1845, 10 Oct 1845; *Hobart Town Courier* 24 Apr 1830; *The Standard* 7 Mar 1837 p. 1; *Courier* 30 Jul 1845, 27 Sep 1845, 15 Sep 1847; *Morning Chronicle* 16 Oct 1845; *Sydney Morning Herald* 20 Aug 1847; *Hobart Mercury* 7 Jan 1862—**TAHO:** CON 40-1-1 p. [160]; CON 19-1-13 p. 135; CSO 26-1-1 p. 249 index to Folio 7505 in CSO 24.

8 Diamonds - Mary Ann Cummings

Newspapers: *Trewman's Exeter Flying Post or Plymouth and Cornish Advertiser* (Exeter, England), 9 Mar 1848, Issue 4291; *Cornwall Chronicle* 24 Sep 1851—**TAHO:** CON 41-1-18 no. 920; CON 15-1-4 pp. 330-331; SC 195-1-31 No. 2808; ADM 101-71 Reel 3211.

9 Diamonds - Mary Braid

BDM (TAHO): RGD 34-1-2 Burial Campbell Town 1340/1844—**Newspapers:** *Caledonian Mercury* 24 Aug 1833, 30 Jan 1834, 13 Feb 1834, 15 Feb 1834; *Colonial Times* 31 Oct 1843 p. 4; *The Cornwall Chronicle* 11 Oct 1845 p. 241—**NRS:** AD14-34-361; JC26-1834-354 (Courtesy A Davidson)—**TAHO:** CON 40-1-1 p. 161; CON 31-1-5 p. 346—**Web:** http://digital.nls.uk/broadsides/broadside. cfm/id/14648; http://www.familysearch.com (baptismal records of Scotland); http://www. environment.gov.au/cgi-bin/ahdb/search. pl?mode=place_detail;place_id=10872; http://www.orphanschool.org.au/showorphan.php?orphan_ID=438.

10 Diamonds - Ellen Bercary

BDM (TAHO): RGD 37-1-12 Marriage Hobart 317/1853—**Newspapers:** *The Argus* 19 Aug 1876 p.10, 6 Oct 1876 p. 6, 9 Oct 1876 p. 7—**TAHO:** CON 41-1-12 no. 825; CON 15-1-4 pp. 44-45; CON 138-1-1 pp.11-12 no.4; CON 52-1-6; CON 33-1-72 no.16799; CON 14-1-32 pp. 48-49; CON 18-1-44; CB 713-1-1 p. 148.

Jack of Diamonds - Rosannah MacDowell and Sarah Stanhope

BDM (TAHO): RGD 33-1-1 Birth Hobart 836/1842; RGD 33-1-1 Birth Hobart 837/1842; RGD 33-1-1 Birth Hobart 838/1842; RGD 35-1-41 Death Gordon 168/1872—**Books:** Tardif 1990 pp. 1559-1560—**Misc:** Baring-Gould 1877—**Newspapers:** *Lancaster Gazette and General Advertiser* 27 Mar 1813; *Hull Packet and Original Weekly Commercial, Literary and General Advertiser* 24 Aug 1813, 22 May 1827, 22 Jan 1828, 18 Jul 1834, 19 Sep 1834; *Morning Chronicle* 22 Jan 1819; *Bristol Mercury* 25 Jan 1819; *York Herald, and General Advertiser* 26 Apr 1823; *Hobart Town Gazette* 15 Jul 1826, 14 Apr 1827, 7 Jul 1827; *Colonial Times* 22 Jun 1827; *Sydney Gazette* Jul, Aug 1827; 11 Feb 1834; *Morning Post* 24 Jan 1828; *Standard* (London) 24 Jan 1828; *Barrow's Worcester Journal* 14 Feb 1828; *Hobart Town Courier* 28 Jun 1828, 10 Mar 1858; *Manchester Times* 10 Nov 1852; 19 Mar 1853—**SRNSW:** NSW musters of convicts 1823, 1824, 1825—**TAHO:** CON 40-1-7 p. 46; CON 40-1-9 p. 67; CON 31-1-9 p. 112; CSO 1-344-7875 p. 119; CSO 5-86-1885 p. 183; Will of Rosannah McDowell AD 960-1-9; Order no. 152 for admissions to Orphan Schools - SWD 24 p. 123.

Queen of Diamonds - Charlotte Williams

Books: Beddoe 1977 pp. 65-71; Beddoe 1979a pp. 67-74; Beddoe 1979b—**Newspapers:** 'Carmarthen Assizes' *Carmarthen Journal* 22 Jul 1831 p. 3; *Cambrian* 6 Aug 1831 p. 1; *Staffordshire Gazette* 13 Aug 1831 p. 4; *Morning Post* (London, England) 15 Aug 1831; *Chester Courant* 16 Aug 1831 p. 4; *Berrow's Worcester Journal* (Worcester, England) 18 Aug 1831; *Worcester Journal* 18 Aug 1831 p. 4; *Belfast News-Letter* (Belfast, Ireland) 19 Aug 1831; *Newcastle Courant* (Newcastle-upon-Tyne, England) 20 Aug 1831; *Leamington Spa Courier* 20 Aug 1831 p. 1; *Devizes and Wiltshire Gazette* 1 Sep 1831 p. 1—**SRNSW:** Ticket of Leave for James

Williams – 4-4156 reel 942; Conditional Pardon recommended for James Williams 4-44800 reel 798—**TAHO**: CON 40-1-9 p. 337; CON 19-1-12 p. 481; CON 31-1-46 p. 165—**TNA**: Prison Hulk Registers and Letter books 1802-49, UK Public Records Office.

King of Diamonds - Julia, Elizabeth and Emily Salt

BDM (LMA): St Giles-without-Cripplegate, Register of Baptism, P69-GIS-A01-Ms 6423, item 3; Info. leaflet no. 59: *Prison Records*, published Mar 2011—**BDM (TAHO)**: RGD 35-1-29 Death New Norfolk 822/1860—**Misc**: Correspondence between Secretary of State for the Colonies and the Lt. Governor of Van Diemen's Land on the Subject of Convict Discipline, Colonial Office, Downing Street, 1846; England & Wales, Death Index, 1837-1915 vol. 1d, p. 50; Harris Family Tree courtesy of Shirley Harris, East Bentleigh, Victoria—**TNA**: 1841 England Census - Class HO 107 - Piece 708, Book 5, St Leonard Shoreditch Civil Parish, Middlesex, Enumeration District 18, folio 28, p. 15, line 7, GSU roll 438818—**Web**: http://www.stgilesnewsite.co.uk/history/.

Ace of Diamonds - Isabella Boswell

Misc: BPP 1869, p. 62—**TAHO**: CON 41-1-31 no. 1129; CON 15-1-7 pp. 77-78; CON 19-1-9.

SPADES

2 Spades - Sarah Hughes

BDM (TAHO): RGD 33-1-32 Birth Campbell Town 158/1854; RGD 35-1-3 Death Hobart 254/1850—**Books**: Bateson 1983, pp. 369, 393; Brand 1990 p. 204—**TAHO**: CON 41-1-11 no. 655; CON 15-1-4 pp. 14-15—**TNA**: HO 18-172-17 Criminal Petitions Series II.

3 Spades - Susanna Webb

BDM (TAHO): RGD 34-1-1 Burial Hobart 4393/1836; RGD 37-1-1 Marriage Hobart 576/1840—**Misc**: Midlands Trade Directories 1770-1941 - Midlands Historical Data, Solihull, West Midlands—**Newspapers**: *Colonial Times* 23 Sep 1851; *Mercury* 9 May 1855; *Birmingham Daily Post* 25 Feb 1858 Issue 60, 3 Dec 1858 p. 2, issue 259; *Courier* 18 Feb 1859 p. 3—**TAHO**: CON 40-1-10 p. 177, POL 220-1-1 p. 62; POL 220-1-2 p. 221.

4 Spades - Mary Pullen

Books: *Australian Dictionary of Biography* 1966 p.77; Damousi 1997 p. 39; Nicholson 1983, p. 152; Stanhope n.d.—**CCC**: Trial of Mary Pullen (t18280529-72)—**TAHO**: CON 40-1-7 p. [32]; CON 19-1-13; CSO 95-1-1 p. 27; ADM 101-32 Reel 3197.

5 Spades - Eliza McIntyre

Newspapers: *Colonial Times* 9 Oct 1855 pp. 2-3; *Hobart Town Mercury* 10 Oct 1855 pp. 2-3; *Hobart Town Daily Mercury* 2 Feb 1858 p. 21, Jun 1859 p. 3—**TAHO**: CON 41-1-7 no. 594 and 2 subsequent pages; CON 15-1-3 pp. 200-201.

6 Spades - Elizabeth Mack

BDM (TAHO): RGD 37-1-14 Marriage New Norfolk 1065/1855—**Books**: Bateson 1983 pp. 370-371; Damousi 1997 pp. 67, 69; Hawkings 2009 p. 72—**Misc**: BPP 1869, pp. 56, 64, 70—**TAHO**: CON 41-1-25 no. 1067; CON 15-1-6 pp. 76-77; CON 52-1-7 pp. 36 & 38.

7 Spades - Biddy Yack McKenna
BDM (TAHO): RGD 35-1-6 Death Hobart
4148/1863; RGD 35-1-7 Death Hobart
7492/1868—TAHO: CON 41-1-5 no. 562;
CON 15-1-3 pp. 116-117; CON 19-1-4;
CON 52-1-7 p. 458; CON 138-1-1 pp.
153-154.

8 Spades - Sarah BROMLEY
BDM (TAHO): RGD 37-1-3 Marriage
Hobart 414/1843—**Books:** Bateson 1983
pp. 360-361, 386; Heard 1981 p. 158;
MacDonald 2005 p. 75; Nicholson 1983;
Pope [1990] p. 152—**Newspapers:** Hobart Town
Courier 28 Feb 1829, 21 Jan 1832, 24 Aug
1832, 3 Apr 1835; Colonial Times 15 Jun 1831—
TAHO: CON 40-1-1 p. 74; CON 19-1-13;
CON 31-1-38 p. 295; CSO 1-368-8375.

9 Spades - Elizabeth May
Books: Hardy 1985; Tardif 1990 pp. 57-
59—**Misc:** NSW Australian Convict Registers
of Conditional and Absolute Pardons Fiche
3164, 4/1846 p.76—**TAHO:** CON 40-1-7
p. 49—**Web:** http://www.windsorcyclists.
org.au/index.php/42-about-windsor-cy-
clists/10-our-logo [accessed Jan 2014].

10 Spades - Margaret HAINES
Books: Daniels 1998 p. 228; Mayhew 1968
p. 359—**CCC:** Trial of Margaret Haines
(t18490917-1830)—**Misc:** BPP 1869, p.
302—**Newspapers:** Hobart Town Daily 20 Mar
1858 p. 3; Courier 22 Oct 1858, p. 3; Mercury
1 Dec 1858 p. 2—**TAHO:** CON 41-1-25 no.
805; CON 42-1-1 p. 30; CON 15-1-6 pp.
68-69; CON 138-2-1 pp. 75, 166.

Jack of Spades - Mary Devereux
CCC: Trial of Mary Devereux (t18310217-
9)—**Misc:** Registration of deaths, G&K
502898—**TAHO:** CON 40-1-3 p. 67;
CON 19-1-13; SWD 28-1-1; CSO 24-190-
6979.

Queen of Spades - Mary Hickey
Newspapers: Mercury 24 Jan 1878 p. 2, 4 Jun
1878 p. 2, 10 Oct 1878 p. 2, 29 Apr 1879
p. 2, 16 May 1879 p. 2, 21 May 1879 p. 2, 1
Dec 1880 p. 2, 8 Dec 1880 p. 4—**TAHO:**
CON 41-1-33, no. 917; CON 15-1-7 pp.
215-216; CON 19-1-10.

King of Spades - Anne Lovell
Books: Rayner 1981; Skemp 1967—**Newspapers:** Hobart Town Gazette and Van Diemen's Land
Advertiser 2 May 1823 p. 2, 4 Oct 1823 p. 3,
25 Oct 1823, p. 3; Colonial Times 14 Sep 1827
pp. 2-3, 7 Sep 1831 pp. 3-4, 5 Oct 1831
p. 3; Hobart Town Courier 10 Oct 1829 p. 4—
Web: 'Lovell, Esh (1796–1865)'. Australian
Dictionary of Biography, National Centre
of Biography, Australian National University, http://adb.anu.edu.au/biography/
lovell-esh-2374/text3121 [accessed 12 May
2014].

Ace of Spades - Margaret Dalzeil
BDM (TAHO): RGD 32-1-4 Birth
Launceston 5731/1862; RGD 32-1-4 Birth
Launceston 5732/1862; RGD 33-1-40
Birth Launceston 128/1862; RGD 35-1-54
Death Launceston 230/1885; RGD 37-1-17
Marriage Launceston 601/1858—**Books:**
Bateson 1983 p. 37; Lord 1992—**Newspa-
pers:** Cornwall Chronicle 28 Jun 1871 p. 3, 17
Apr 1872 p. 3; Launceston Examiner 20 Apr
1872 p. 2, 17 Jul 1885 p. 3 c. 6—**TAHO:**
CON 41-1-31 no. 780; CON 15-1-7 pp.
87-88; CON 52-1-6; CON 52-1-7 p. 72;
CON 138-2-1 pp. 40, 41, 43, 44, 48, 192,
209.

BIBLIOGRAPHY

Abbott, F. & Hall, E. S. 1865, *Meteorology records and analysis of the observatory records for April 1865 in conjunction with those of births and deaths.* Monthly Notices of Papers & Proceedings of the Royal Society of Tasmania, Hobart.

Australian Dictionary of Biography – Vol. 1, 1788-1850, A-H. 1966, Melbourne University Press, Carlton, Vic.

Baring-Gould, S.1877, *"Snowden Dunhill – the convict"(S. Baring-Gould, published 1877). A summary presentation of "The life of Snowden Dunhill, as told by himself" (S. Dunning aka Dunhill, published 1834)* (online). https://archive.org/details/TheLifeOfSnowdenDunhillAsToldByHimself [accessed 13 May 2014].

Bateson, C. 1983, *The convict ships, 1787-1868.* Library of Australian History, Sydney.

Beddoe, D. 1977, Carmarthenshire women and criminal transportation to Australia 1787-1852. In *The Carmarthenshire Antiquary*, XIII.

Beddoe, D. 1979a, Carmarthenshire's convict women in nineteenth-century Van Diemen's Land. In *The Carmarthenshire Antiquary*, XV.

Beddoe, D. 1979b, *Welsh convict women: A study of women transported from Wales to Australia 1787–1852,* Stewart William, Barry, Wales.

Brand, I. 1990, *The convict probation system: Van Diemen's Land, 1839-1854.* Blubberhead Press, Hobart.

[BPP]. 1969, *Correspondence on the subject of convict discipline and transportation 1852-53: Crime and punish-ment: Transportation.* (British Parliamentary Papers: vol. 12). Irish University Press, Shannon, Ireland.

Chick, N. 2009, Applications by convicts for permission to marry. In *Tasmanian Ancestry* 30 (3), Dec.

Cowley, T. & Snowden, D. 2013, *Patchwork prisoners: The Rajah quilt and the women who made it.*

Research Tasmania, Hobart.

Coxe, J. R.1825, *The American dispensatory containing the natural, chemical, pharmaceutical and medical history of the different substances employed in medicine,* J.R.A. Skerrett, Philadelphia.

Damousi, J. 1997, *Depraved and disorderly: Female convicts, sexuality and gender in colonial Australia.* Cambridge University Press, Melbourne.

Daniels, K. 1998, *Convict women.* Allen & Unwin, St. Leonards, NSW.

Elias, P. & A. (eds.). 2003, *A few from afar: Jewish lives in Tasmania from 1804.* The Hobart Hebrew Congregation, Hobart.

Female Convicts Research Centre, 2014. *Female Convicts in Van Diemen's Land* (database).

Frost, L. 2001, Eliza Churchill tells... In *Chain letters: Narrating convict lives.* L. Frost & H. Maxwell-Stewart (eds.). Melbourne University Press.

Frost, L. (ed.). 2011, *Convict lives at the Ross Female Factory.* Convict Women's Press, Hobart.

Frost, L. 2012, *Abandoned women: Scottish convicts exiled beyond the seas.* Allen & Unwin, Sydney.

Frost, L. 2013, "At home" on a mission station and in a Female Factory: imagining Mary Hutchinson. In *Empire calling: Administer-ing colonial Australasia and India,* eds. R. Crane, A. Johnston, and C. Vijayasree. Cambridge University Press (India).

Goc, N. 2013, Infanticide in the Van Diemen's Land Press. In *Women, Infanticide and the Press 1822-1922.* Ashgate, Burlington, VT.

Grundy, J. E. 2006, *A dictionary of medical & related terms for the family historian.* Swansong Publications, Rotherham, South Yorks.

Gunson, N. 1967, Oakes, Francis (1770-1844). In *Australian dictionary of biography,* ed. D. Pike. Melbourne University Press, vol. 2.

Hardy, B. 1985, *Early Hawkesbury settlers.* Kangaroo Press, Kenthurst, NSW.

Hawkings, D. 2009, *Criminal ancestors: A guide to historical criminal records in England and Wales.* History Press, Stroud, Gloucs.

Heard, D. 1981, *The journal of Charles O'Hara Booth: Commandant of the Port Arthur penal settlement.* Tasmanian Historical Research Association, Hobart.

Hutchinson, R. C. 1961, The Reverend John Hutchinson. In *Papers and Proceedings of the Tasmanian Historical Research Association* 9(3).

Hutchinson, R. C. 1965, Mrs Hutchinson and the Female Factories of early Australia. In *Papers and Proceedings of the Tasmanian Historical Research Association* 11(2).

Levy, M. C. I. 1953, *Governor George Arthur: A colonial benevolent despot.* Georgian House, Great Britain.

Lord, R. 1992, *Impression Bay: Convict probation station to civilian quarantine station: Being the story of the fever immigrant ship Persian along with her passengers quarantined at Impression Bay, Tasman's Peninsula in 1857.* R. Lord and Partners, Taroona, Tas.

MacDonald, H. 2005, Dissecting Mary McLauchlan. In *Human remains: Episodes in human dissection.* Melbourne University Press.

MacDonald, H. P. 2006, *Human remains: Dissection and its histories.* Yale University Press, New Haven, Conn.

Mayhew, H. 1968, *London labour and the London poor.* Vol. IV. Dover Publications, New York.

Melville, H. 1833, *Van Diemen's Land: Comprehending a variety of information likely to be interesting to the emigrant.* Henry Melville, Hobart Town.

Nicholson, I. H. 1983, *Shipping arrivals and departures, Tasmania vol. 1, 1803-1833.* Roebuck Society, Canberra.

Phillips, W. 1855, *The wild tribes of London.* Ward and Lock, London.

Pope, T. [1990], *Irish freemasonry in Tasmania* (online). http://www.irishmasonichistory. com/uploads/1/0/3/8/10381775/irish_free-masonry_in_tasmania_by_w.bro._tony_pope. pdf [accessed 28 Mar 2014].

Purtscher, J. 1994, *Apprentices and absconders from Queen's Orphanage, Hobart Town, 1860-1883.* Irene Schaffer, New Town, Tas.

Rayner, T. 1981, *Historical survey of the Female Factory Historic Site, Cascades, Hobart.* (Occasional Paper: no. 3). National Parks and Wildlife Service, Tasmania, Hobart.

Rosner, L. 2010, *The anatomy murders: Being the true and spectacular history of Edinburgh's notorious Burke and Hare.* University of Pennsylvania Press, Philadelphia.

Snowden, D. 2005, "A white rag burning": Irish women who committed arson in order to be transported to Van Diemen's Land. PhD thesis, University of Tasmania.

Stanhope, Charles [1753-1829] (online). *Old Dictionary of National Biography* (DNB). Oxford University Press. http://www.oxforddnb. com/templates/olddnb.jsp?articleid=26242 [accessed Mar 2014].

Stringer, R. G. 1885, *A pioneer: A memoir of the Rev. John Thomas, missionary to the Friendly islands.* T. Woolmer, London.

Tardif, P. 1990, *Notorious strumpets and dangerous girls: Convict women in Van Diemen's Land 1803-1829.* Angus & Robertson, North Ryde, NSW.

Williams, J. 1994, *Ordered to the island: Irish convicts and Van Diemen's Land.* Crossing Press, Sydney.

Wright, D. & Clancy, E. G. 1993, *The Methodists: A history of Methodism in New South Wales.* Allen & Unwin, St Leonards, NSW.